The Clinician's Guide to Medical Writing

The Clinician's Guide to Medical Writing

Robert B. Taylor, M.D.

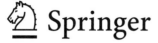 Springer

Robert B. Taylor, M.D.
Department of Family Medicine
Mail Code FM
Oregon Health & Science Univ. School of Medicine
Portland, Oregon 97239-3098, USA
taylorr@ohsu.edu

CIP data available upon request.

ISBN 0-387-22249-9 Printed on acid-free paper.

Printed in the United States of America. (GP/EB)

9 8 7 6 5 4 3 2 1 SPIN 10985809

springeronline.com

This book is dedicated to two mentors who have been important in my life:

Martha E. Irwin, my Latin and Spanish teacher, who taught me to value words and their meanings,

and

Charles F. Visokay, M.D., my first medical editor, who helped me learn how to write for clinicians.

Preface

This book is for the clinician who wants to write. It is for the physician, physician assistant, or nurse practitioner who sees patients and who wants to contribute to the medical literature. You may be an assistant professor aspiring to promotion or a clinician in private practice who seeks the personal enrichment that writing can bring. If you are new to medical writing or even if you have been the author of some articles or book chapters and seek to improve your abilities, this book can help you.

Who am I that I can make this assertion and write this book, both fairly presumptuous? Here's my reasoning. As a practicing physician, writing has been my avocation; unlike the authors of many other writing books, I am not a journal editor. Over 14 years in private practice and 26 years in academic medicine, I have written all the major models described in this book: review articles, case reports, editorials, letters to the editor, book reviews, book chapters, edited books, authored books, and reports of clinical research studies. Most have been published. Not all. Perhaps my most significant qualification is not that I have managed to produce a lengthy curriculum vitae. In my opinion, what is more important for you, the reader, is that I have made all the errors. That's right, the mistakes. Over the years, I have jumbled spelling, mixed metaphors, tangled syntax, gotten lost in my own outline, written on unimportant topics, and submitted articles to the wrong journals. But along the way, I have published 22 medical books and several hundred papers and book chapters in the literature. This book is written to share what I have learned—what works and what doesn't in medical writing.

This book is intended to help clinicians translate their practice observations and ideas into written form and eventually into print. In striving to achieve this purpose, I have written the book with four objectives in mind. These objectives are to help the clinician-writer

- understand more about the art of medical writing, including motivation, conceptualization, mechanics, and frustrations;
- discover how to write in the different models found in the medical literature, including review articles, case reports, editorials, letters, book chapters, research papers, and more;
- learn how to get a manuscript published; and
- recognize that writing can be fun.

The book's 10 chapters cover basic concepts in medical writing and how to write various types of articles and book chapters. The content is a blend of personal experience and research on the Web and in printed sources. Throughout all chapters, I have attempted to follow the time-honored principle of supporting theory with examples, some from actual published materials and some created to help illustrate the ideas presented.

In Chapter 1, I challenge authors to consider three questions before beginning work on an article or book: *So what? Who cares? Where will it be published?* As the author, I believe that I should answer the three questions in regard to this book. The "So what?" question asks what is new and different, and I think that the answer lies in the fact that I address medical writing knowledge and skills from the viewpoint of the clinician, not that of the medical journal editor or professor of English literature. The "Who cares?" issue concerns the potential reader; for this book, that is the clinician who writes for the medical literature. In response to the "Where will it be published?" question, I am pleased that this book is published by Springer-Verlag, the world's leading publisher of scientific books, with whom I have had an author–publisher relationship since 1976.

As a clinician, you have a tremendous source for writing ideas—the patients you see each day. Think about the meaning of a cluster of uncommon problems you have observed recently, the unlikely manifestation of a common disease, or the extraordinary courage displayed by one of your patients.

Perhaps you have found a new way to use an old remedy, or you have your own thoughts about a recently published study. This book is about helping you—the practicing clinician—recognize the reportable idea and *write it up*.

Happy writing!

Portland, Oregon   Robert B. Taylor, M.D.
May 2004

Table of Contents

Dedication   v
Preface   vii
About This Book   xiii

1   Getting Started in Medical Writing   1

2   Basic Writing Skills   29

3   From Page One to the End   61

4   Technical Issues in Medical Writing   85

5   What's Special About Medical Writing?   105

6   How to Write a Review Article   127

7   Case Reports, Editorials, Letters to the Editor,
Book Reviews, and Other Publication Models   143

8   Writing Book Chapters and Books   167

9   How to Write a Report of a Clinical Study   195

10   Getting your Writing Published   213

Appendix 1   Glossary of Terms Used in Medical
Writing   247

Appendix 2   Commonly Used Proofreader's Marks   253

Appendix 3   Commonly Used Medical Abbreviations   255

Appendix 4   Normal Laboratory Values for
Adult Patients   259

Index   263

About This Book

> True ease in writing comes from art, not chance,
> As those move easiest who have learn'd to dance.
>
> Alexander Pope

After reading this book, you will have a better understanding of the art of writing, both of writing in general and, specifically, of medical writing, with all its idiosyncrasies. This short introduction tells a little about the book's organization and its own peculiarities, including word use, reference style, and the examples and allusions you will encounter. In the end, our common goal is to find some true ease in writing, through consideration of both theory and examples from the literature, and by looking at what constitutes good and not-so-good writing.

The book progresses from the theoretical to the practical. It begins with basic writing topics and skills. Next comes a consideration of the various models for medical writing, from review article to report of a research study. The final chapter discusses how to get your work into print. The appendix has some handy tools that may help you along the way, including a glossary of medical writing terms, proofreader's marks, and some tables of commonly used abbreviations and laboratory reference values that you may use in your publications (with attribution, please, but you need not request permission from Springer-Verlag or from me).

In the early chapters on basic writing skills, I use the word *article*, even though we know that later in the book the principles of authorship described will also apply to editorials, letters to the editor, and research reports. In using words, I will often go to the Greek or Latin roots; doing so helps me use words more precisely.

Within chapters, you will also note some reference citations in parentheses. These are used for articles and books that are the sources of writing examples. Although I believe it unlikely that any reader would actually want to consult these writings, I have provided abbreviated citations, just in case.

At the end of each chapter are references presented in the style of the Uniform Requirements for Manuscripts Submitted to Biomedical Journals, a very useful guide that will be discussed in later chapters. Using this reference style for the book models the way you will generally prepare citations for your medical articles.

I have done my best to make this book a pleasure to read. This includes using short, strong words, and, at times, colorful images. I have included allusions to medical history, classical writing, mystery novels, popular songs, opera, and movies. We will visit Pogo and Snoopy, zombies and clones, Billy Crystal and Frau Röntgen, Princess Turandot and Yogi Berra. As you read along you will also learn some medical information, such as whether or not flu vaccine can prevent ear infection in children and whether continuity of care can lower health care costs. All the examples in the book help illustrate points about medical writing that I consider important.

My wife, Anita D. Taylor, M.A. Ed., has read every word in this book at least twice and has provided ideas that are reflected in what you will read. For her contributions, I am truly grateful.

I hope that what follows will help you master the art of writing, to "move easiest" by learning—not really new dance steps—but some helpful tips on how to walk the path from idea to print.

1

Getting Started in Medical Writing

Does being a clinician make you or me a capable medical writer? No, it doesn't, any more than being a physician qualifies me to be a good stock picker, business manager, or even vacation planner. It only means that I have medical knowledge and skills, and am trained to care for patients. On the other hand, just because you are a clinician who sees patients daily does not mean that you cannot become a capable, even great, writer. Being that great writer requires knowledge, skill, experience, the capacity to endure rejection, and a strong will to succeed.

The knowledge part includes both medical and "writing" knowledge. Let us assume that, by virtue of your clinical practice, you have the medical knowledge. Then what you must master are the body of information and the technical skills that can help you become a great writer. You must know how to assemble and use basic writing resources. You also need to understand key issues in medical writing such as how to get started and how to get finished, the various models of medical writing, how to prepare a manuscript, and how to get your work published. Acquiring this knowledge is no small task, but it can be done.

Writing for the medical literature has its own special considerations. Writing vibrant prose is not usually the key issue, and at times may appear to be disadvantageous. Rew[1] has written, "A fog has settled on scientific English. Well-written English effortlessly communicates the writer's intent to the reader. Unfortunately, far too often, science is written in a form that renders the content hard to understand, and which makes unreasonable demands on the reader." It seems that many medical articles, notably reports of clinical research studies, are written to be published and cited, but not to be read. I hope that you and I can aspire to a higher level of writing skill, and that editors and readers will appreciate the enhanced readability of our work.

The ability to endure rejection is a must. I began medical writing in the early 1970s while in small-town private practice. I had some early success in conducting clinical studies and seeing the results in print in respected journals. I also wrote some articles for controlled circulation, advertiser-supported journals. Not everything I wrote was published. I also began writing health books for nonmedical people, what the editors call the "lay audience." Here I collected so many rejection letters that I could have wallpapered a room with them. Only when I began writing and editing medical books did my acceptance rate become favorable. However, after 30 years of medical writing experience, I still receive rejections for clinical papers, editorials, and book proposals. And, yes, it still hurts.

If you aspire to be a medical writer you will need determination. Being a writer takes a lot of work and you really need to want it. But if you develop the itch to write, it can only be relieved by the scratch of the pen—or today by the click of the computer keyboard. If you begin to see yourself as a writer working on a project, as I am working on this book today, then you will think about the project whenever you have a spare moment, and as ideas occur, you will jot them on a scrap of paper, index card, or personal digital assistant. You will record the concept or phrase when and where you can, just so it doesn't get away, because that is what writers do.

WHY WE WRITE

For years I have periodically conducted writing workshops for clinicians. Conducting writing workshops, of course, guarantees an audience that is self-selected to be more interested in writing than those in competing workshops on how to perform a better hemorrhoidectomy or how to manage one's office practice. Generally, most of the participants are previously published medical authors, at least to some degree. Each of these workshops begins with the same question: Why do we write? The answers, while diverse, tend to be the same in each workshop, and are listed in Table 1.1. I am going to discuss a few of these.

First, let's discuss and dismiss the final entry on the list—earn income. Medical writing is not lucrative.

TABLE 1.1.   Reasons why we write

Gain intellectual stimulation
Share ideas
Report research
Express an opinion
Generate discussion
Advance one's discipline
Assert "ownership" of a topic
Attain promotion/tenure
Report a case
Enhance one's personal reputation
Achieve some small measure of immortality by publishing our ideas
Earn income

Advertiser-supported publications (more about them later) often pay a few hundred dollars for an article. Book royalties are generally meager; after all, the audience of clinicians who might buy your book is small. Book chapters, editorial, and research reports pay nothing and are written for other reasons. If your goal is wealth, you should add more clinical hours to your schedule or buy stocks that go up—anything but medical writing.

What about the other reasons? For those in academic medicine, promotion and tenure are very important, and publications are the key to success. As medical schools become increasingly dependent on clinicians seeing patients for economic survival, it would seem that this clinical effort would be rewarded with the carrots of career achievement—promotion to the next rank and, where applicable, tenured faculty positions. In 1988, a study at Johns Hopkins Medical School reported, "Those who were promoted had had about twice as many articles published in peer-reviewed journals as those who were not promoted."[2] I have not seen a recent similar study, but my academic colleagues do not tell me that anything has changed, and an academic faculty member who bets his or her career on advancement without publications is taking a dangerous path. Yet some seem to be doing so.

I tell young faculty that, as a broad generalization, it takes at least two publications a year to be considered as "satisfactory" in scholarly activity when it comes time for promotion.

Some can be clinical reviews or case reports, but others must be research reports published in refereed journals. Also, you must be the first author on your share of the papers, not always second or third author. Faculty members who chiefly see patients often do not get this message. A 2003 paper by Beasley and Wright[3] surveyed faculty in 80 medical schools in 35 states. They differentiated between clinician investigators (the research faculty) and clinician educators (the patient care faculty) and concluded, "Clinician educators are less familiar with promotion guidelines, meet less often with superiors for performance review, and have less protected time than clinician investigator colleagues."

In my opinion the most enduring reason to be a medical writer is the intellectual stimulation. Medical writers have a lot of fun learning about their topics, rummaging in their imaginations for the best way to present material, and finding just the right words to say what is important. They stimulate discussion. For example, last month I published an article on leadership with the premise that leadership skills can be learned. A reader disagreed, stating that my article had "missed the mark" and that the top leaders have inherited abilities and character traits. I had an enjoyable time composing my reply.

There is also the pleasant side effect of getting known. As an editor of a number of medical reference books, I have had the wonderful experience of visiting clinics in Asia, Europe, and South America, and having young doctors exclaim, "Doctor Taylor, I have read your book." On a practical level, if you are a referral physician who specializes in, for example, refractive surgery of the eye or the management of Parkinson's disease, publishing articles on these topics helps assure referrals.

In the end, however, when the going gets tough, and your paper has been rejected again, what will sustain you is not the discussion with readers, the recognition, or the referrals. It is the simple joy of writing.

WHY WE DON'T WRITE

If writing is such a joy, why don't we write? And for those in academic medicine and whose career advancement

TABLE 1.2. Reasons given for not writing

Not enough time
Nothing to write about
No one to work with in writing
Lack of secretarial support
Lack of knowledge as to how to research information
No mentor for writing activities
No motivation
No self-confidence
Don't know how to start
"I hate writing!"

depends on publications, it is curious that so many resist writing.

In my workshops on medical writing, the second discussion question is "Why don't we write?" Table 1.2 lists some of the answers received over the years.

What about the resource issues in the list above? Time to write is always mentioned early in the discussion. No one in private practice has revenue-generating time that is allocated to writing. Those in academic practice soon find that they don't either. For academicians, time to do research and to write must be "bought" by obtaining funding (which is why grant writing is important). For the rest of us, writing time is going to be carved out of personal time. When I was in private solo practice, my writing time was in the early morning, before breakfast and when my family was asleep. For others, the time will be weekend mornings or late at night. In workshops, sometimes I have encountered vocal—sometimes even angry—disagreement with my "writing on your own time" beliefs, but most experienced medical writers and editors will tell you this is the way it is.

Whatever time you designate as writing time must be vigorously protected. In practice patients will get sick and call; this is the virtue of writing in the early morning or late-night hours when the telephone is quiet. In academic medicine, you may need to close the door while writing or go to the library, to prevent colleagues from coming to discuss problem residents, curriculum changes, or patient referrals—anything but writing.

How about the lack of ideas, lack of secretarial support, lack of colleagues, and so forth? Any clinician seeing 15 to 25 patients a day encounters a wide variety of clinical phenomena that could present the idea for an article: common causes of pelvic pain, ways to manage the patient with a low back strain, an unusual manifestation of lupus erythematosus, herbal therapy in the treatment of depression, and much more. The variety you see depends on your specialty. Your writing ideas will come from your clinical encounters. This is as it should be, because it brings immediacy to your writing and provides the credibility you need to write on the topic. Later in the book, we will discuss how to develop clinical observations into writing topics, outlines, and articles.

In my opinion, laments about lack of secretarial help, collegial support, and research access are not as valid as they once were. Why? Because of the computer and the Internet. As recently as 5 or 6 years ago, I was highly dependent on secretarial support; I dictated my articles and made corrections by hand to be changed on computer. Today I use the Microsoft Word program on my computer, doing most of the typing myself; the computer's efficiency has led me to change my writing methods. With e-mail, coauthors are also readily available. In fact, I can pass documents back and forth with colleagues across the country by e-mail just as readily as with those down the hall.

The World Wide Web has revolutionized research, making information needed for writing readily available to anyone with a computer and Internet access. Because knowing how to use the available resources is so important to medical writers, we will shortly spend time learning about what is online and how to use it. Basically, you can find out about anything that you need to know while sitting at your desk, if only you learn how to do it.

The lack of self-confidence is quickly overcome after a few publications, which may also help to spark motivation.

Regarding the last entry on Table 1.2, I can't do much for those who really hate to write.

RANDOM THOUGHTS ABOUT MEDICAL WRITING

Writing as History

In 1912 the citizens of the village of Caledonia, New York, placed a large boulder as a monument commemorating the historic treaty between Chief Ganaiodia, representing the Native Americans in the area, and the local villagers and farmers. As a civic leader, my grandmother had an idea. She dispatched my mother, age 9, to the grocery store to buy a tin of cookies. Yes, those were the days that cookies came in tin boxes and one could safely send a 9-year-old child alone to the grocery store. When my mother returned, grandmother removed the cookies, which I am sure were put to good use. What she wanted was the box, into which she placed several items, including a copy of the village weekly newspaper. The box was then buried beneath the boulder as a time capsule. I believe that it is still there beneath the boulder.

Your writing is a time capsule. It shows what you and your colleagues think today about important issues such as diagnosis, treatment, prevention, prognosis, health policy, practice management, and much more. As readers we use medical writing to take looks back in history.

Let us look at the historic figures in medicine. Who comes to mind? Hippocrates, Galen, Maimonides, Paracelsus, Vesalius, Harvey, Osler, and more. (I am sure that, in choosing just a few to discuss briefly, I have omitted many favorites, but I am going to try to make a point). Three hundred years before the Common Era (CE), Hippocrates wrote *On Hemorrhoids*, *On Fractures*, *On Ulcers*, *On the Surgery*, *On the Sacred Disease*, and the *Book of Aphorisms*. Galen, writing in Rome during the 2nd century CE, compiled the medical knowledge of the day into an encyclopedic work that endured as an authoritative reference for centuries. Maimonides wrote on diet, reptile poisoning, and asthma during the 12th century CE. Later, during the Renaissance Paracelsus described miner's disease and the treatment of syphilis with mercurials; he gave us the guiding principle of toxicology: "The dose makes the poison." We know this because Paracelsus *wrote* it. Vesalius produced drawings of the body that greatly advanced the study of anatomy. Harvey, in the 1600s, wrote describing the circulation of blood in the body and later William Osler's book *The Principles and Practice of Medicine* defined the practice of medicine in the late 19th century.[4]

Do you notice the common theme above? Is my point becoming clear? While all were undoubtedly outstanding physicians of their day, they are remembered because they *wrote*. They recorded their observations and their thoughts. In doing so, they literally helped make the history of medicine. And by writing, they created the building blocks upon which today's house of medicine stands.

You and I can do a little of this, too. At this time, none of us is likely to become the "father of medicine" or the "father of anatomy." Hippocrates and Vesalius hold those titles. But we can add small 21st century building blocks to the house of medicine, while metaphorically adding some of our work to today's time capsule for someone in the future to ponder.

Writing and Reading

Reading goes with writing like ice cream goes with apple pie—one just makes the other better. All writers must read if they are to be any good at medical writing, and you should read diverse items and for various reasons: for information, for ideas, for structure, for style, and for a sense of history.

All physicians need to read the medical literature regularly to stay up to date in their fields; this is part of being a doctor. (Later, in Chapter 3, we will look at how clinicians read the literature). Your journal reading will help build bridges to your own experience.

Writers also read to seek information—often the difference between browsing and hunting. For example, when writing the section above, I needed to read parts of Sebastian's[4] excellent reference book *A Dictionary of the History of Medicine* to learn about Hippocrates, Galen, and Harvey. No, I did not have all the information in my head.

Writers also read for ideas. Again we both browse and hunt. We read to see what ideas others are putting forth. As I write this, some clinical-interest topics include the resurgence of pertussis, the management of breast cancer, the place of herbal remedies in medicine, and how to treat attention deficit/hyperactivity disorder in children and adults. Or one may hunt: Right now I have promised to write an editorial for a journal within the next 2 months, and I am searching for information on the topic I have chosen.

Reading for structure? What does this mean? By this I mean reading articles analytically. When you read an article that you like—because of the writing, not the topic or statistics—go back and reread the article looking at how the author put it together. How was the title composed? How was the abstract constructed? How did the writer organize the information so that it was clearly presented? What tables and illustrations were used, and were they effective, and why were they effective? How many references were included, and what publications were cited? Reread this chapter before going on to Chapter 2 and think about the questions I just asked as they apply to the chapter you are reading. What are the good points and what could I have done better? In short, look at the craftsmanship of the article or book chapter, as well as the message.

Read also for style. Read well-written medical literature. This may be a little hard to find, as refereed journals have increasingly become the repository for published, citable, but barely readable reports of research data. The writing in the *British Medical Journal* is better than most, and some of the best writing in U.S. medical journals is found in editorials and opinion pieces.

Reading for style includes reading nonmedical books, vitally important to those who aspire to be serious writers. Here you can gain a sense of language, grammar and syntax, and the rhythm of words in good literature. I believe that a medical writer should always be reading a nonmedical book. Read some of the classics, such as the grand metaphoric prose of Herman Melville's *Moby Dick*, the powerful, yet spare journalistic style of Ernest Hemingway's *The Old Man and the Sea*, the subtle and complex style of Jane Austen's *Pride and Prejudice*, and the symbolism of Thomas Mann's *The Magic Mountain*. You might also include a Tom Clancy thriller or Patricia Cornwell medical mystery, or a James Michener epic.

You and I can gain a sense of perspective by reading about our heroes and our language. To read a collection of time-capsule items, try to find a copy of R.H. Major's *Classic Descriptions of Disease*.[5] To learn about the words we use, there is no more scholarly book than J.H. Dirckx's *The Language of Medicine*.[6] And one should include a book on the history of our profession such as Roy Porter's *The Greatest Benefit to Mankind*.[7]

Writing and You

Who Writes?

Is there a profile of the medical writer? There is no single "right" type of person who chooses to write. However, there are degrees of "fit" between a person's preferences and characteristics desirable for writing. It goes beyond mere technical skills. Writing may be an opportunity for you to use your talents and give you great satisfaction while others will describe writing as "frustrating" and "stressful." Most importantly, you need to be aware of your own preferences, strengths, and priorities. Psychological inventories, such as the Myers-Briggs Type Indicator (MBTI), have described personality types that tend to be most attracted to writing as being creative, adaptable, and eager to take on new challenges (INFP, ENFP, INTP, ENTP, in MBTI terminology).[8] If you are writing to a deadline, as for books or magazines, your organizational and time management skills are also factors in your potential success.

Writing as Creativity

Whether what you are writing is a compilation of data in a research report, an editorial about a topic that flames your passions, or a new look at how to treat your favorite disease, your writing involves creativity. This means that you are producing something that comes from you, personally, and that did not exist before you made it. I find this both humbling and energizing. In writing this paragraph, I am putting 89 English words together in a way that no one ever did before. This is exciting.

This creativity is what can get the juices flowing. It helps focus your sense of purpose—that writing is important, especially what you are writing now. The creative process is more important than committees, golf, or the crabgrass in the lawn.

Your rewards come when you have finished something and you can say, "This is great, and I created it," and from others reading the results of your creative effort, and sometimes even responding—even when they disagree.

Of course, creativity is also a solitary process. Note that of the great medical writers in history that we discussed earlier, none had a Boswell to record his thoughts. (From your college courses, perhaps you recall James Boswell, the 18th century writer best known for recording the words of Samuel Johnson.) Nor do we find many coauthors. Each did it alone with parchment and quill, paper and pen. Be aware that your medical writing will require hours spent staring into the computer screen and rummaging in books. It will mean overcoming the tendency to talk with colleagues down the hall, go for coffee, chat on the telephone—anything to maintain contact with other humans. So be prepared for quiet time alone with your ideas. However, you may find that your ideas and your creativity are very good company.

Writing Topics and Your Career
If you are in private practice with no aspirations to an academic career or research grant funding, then you might skip this short section. However, if you are a faculty member seeking academic advancement (promotion and tenure) or a research position, the following can be important career advice. Here it is: Find your topic early in your career and stick with it as long as your can. The "career topic" will be what you write about. It will also be the subject of your research, and perhaps why you receive patient referrals. For example, for years I have written on migraine headaches. Clearly because of my writing review articles and book chapters on this topic, I—as a family physician—became a leading headache referral physician in our academic medical center. I received more headache patient referrals than I really wanted, all because of writing on the topic.

Some topics I have seen young academicians developing recently include: a national scorecard on women's health services, health literacy of patients, the impact of high professional liability rates on physician retention, changes in the quality of health services when patients are forced to change doctors, attention deficit/hyperactivity disorder (AD/HD) in adult patients, the integration of complementary/alternative practices into allopathic medicine, the cost efficiency of various health screening methods, and racial or gender disparities in health care. The list of potential topics is endless.

What is important is to identify a topic that energizes you and that has the potential to endure. For example, one could write on a topic of, for example, treatment of Bartholin cyst or infant crib safety, but would soon run out of things to say and articles to write. It is much better to write on a topic of general interest, with evolving research and, if possible, high social relevance. Then, as you write on various facets of the topic in journals and books, you establish your national position as an authority in the field, which is a requirement for promotion to the rank of professor in academic medical centers. So, if possible, find your career topic early and stick with it.

What should you *not* write about? First of all, don't write on topics outside your area of clinical expertise. The psychiatrist probably shouldn't be writing about knee injuries, and the orthopedic surgeon should find a topic other than AD/HD. Also, do not write on a clinical area in which you do not wish to receive referrals and become recognized locally as an expert. I once knew a general internist who wrote a few articles on alcoholism. He was interested in the topic because his father was an alcoholic. Before long his practice was dominated by alcoholic patients, both through referrals by colleagues and then by patients seeking out the local expert on the topic and by attorneys requesting expert testimony. This shift in practice emphasis was not at all what he had planned.

ASSEMBLING YOUR RESOURCES

Because this topic is so important, I am going to devote space to it early in the book. You must not try to write without assembling what you need to write. Without designating a writing area, acquiring books and computer programs, and learning to use key Web sites, a premature foray into writing is likely to cause frustration.

Your Writing Area

What are your logistic requirements for writing? First of all, you will need a comfortable chair and a desk surface. The chair must support your back, and ideally will have a height adjustment that can change if your shoulders start to ache after a few hours of typing. The surface may be the kitchen table, as long as it is well lit and is large enough to accommodate papers, books, computer, and all the rest.

You will need a computer with Internet access. The days of submitting manuscripts on paper are drawing to a close. My latest article submissions have been online, and paper was needed only for author attestations and signatures. My last two books were submitted on computer disks; I mailed some illustrations that would print better from the original documents than had I scanned and sent them by e-mail. For these two books and at the request of the development editors, I also sent paper copies of the manuscript—a bit of a burden since one book had a manuscript of more than 3000 pages. However, I suspect that all copyediting and typesetting were done from the electronic copy, and I am not sure the paper copies were ever used.

The point of the story is that you will need a computer for composition, revision, and submission. At home and work, I use both desktop and notebook computers. I find the desktop computer easier to use for long sessions of typing. The notebook is more convenient when moving work from place to place, and definitely if the computer must be taken into the shop for repair.

You must have a DSL (digital subscriber line), cable modem, or whatever is the latest way to attain high-speed access to the Internet. If you are using a dial-up modem, plan today to enter the 21st century. If your dial-up modem has a dedicated second home telephone line, you can cancel the second line and get a DSL for a small marginal cost. There is only one concern. With the DSL line, you are likely to be "online" more than with a modem, and this makes you more vulnerable to computer viruses and identity theft. For this reason, you need excellent security; I use Norton Internet Security by Symantec, which contains both a personal firewall and antivirus protection. My live updates keep me current. Each time I log on to the Internet, I check to be sure my Internet security is functioning and up to date.

Other items to have handy are a telephone, notepad, pen or pencils, and a cup of your favorite beverage. Add your books, computer programs, and Web sites, and you are good to go.

Books

If I were advising you a decade ago, this section would be much longer. However, the Internet and the availability of useful Web sites have changed how I search for information. With awareness that this list is rather spare, here are some basic books for the medical writer (and reader):

Dictionaries

A medical dictionary is a must. Do not underestimate the value of a good dictionary. For example, I find the dictionary often the best place to look up a newly encountered syndrome or eponymic disease name. There are good dictionary computer programs, discussed below, but sometimes you just need to look it up in a book that can be held in your hand. Two good ones are *Dorland's Medical Dictionary*, published by W.B. Saunders, and *Stedman's Medical Dictionary*, published by Lippincott Williams & Wilkins (LWW). Each has the Greek, Latin, and other derivations of words, a feature that I value. I use Dorland's for two reasons: First of all, I have used various editions of this dictionary since I was an intern and feel comfortable with it, just like being with an old friend. The second and more practical reason is that on my computer is the *Stedman's Electronic Medical Dictionary*, described below. Thus, I have access to two dictionaries that are not duplicates.

Also have available a general dictionary of the English language. Go to your favorite bookstore and select the one that has the right heft and readable type. Again I look for a dictionary that tells the etymologic derivation of words. I am still using one I have had since high school; after all, the words added each year are probably not new to me. Good dictionaries available today are *Random House Webster's College*

Dictionary (published by Random House) and the *American Heritage Dictionary of the English Language* (published by Houghton Mifflin).

Basic Specialty-Specific Medical Reference Book

Every medical writer needs a basic reference book in his or her specialty. Each specialty has at least two such books. In internal medicine, for example, the basic reference books are Harrison's *Principles of Internal Medicine* (published by McGraw-Hill), Cecil *Essentials of Medicine* (published by W.B. Saunders), and Kelley's *Textbook of Internal Medicine* (published by Lippincott Williams & Wilkins). This gives you a chance to check your clinical data and recommendations against what's generally accepted in the field. Of course, a textbook begins to go out of date as soon as the ink on the pages is dry, and you should make a commitment to buy each new edition as it is released. Still, you will find your omnibus specialty reference book very important to have at hand when needed.

Inter-Specialty Reference Books

The *5-Minute Clinical Consult*, published by Lippincott Williams & Wilkins, is a very useful reference for a wide variety of clinical conditions. Using an outline format, this "cookbook" tells what the busy clinician needs to know about a wide variety of diseases, with an emphasis on the outpatient setting. There is a version that can be loaded onto your personal digital assistant.

The *Quick Look Drug Book* is one of my favorites. Like several of the books noted above, Lippincott Williams & Wilkins publishes it. It is a paperback book, published annually, that is useful for checking drug generic names, brand names, and doses. The latter is vitally important for accuracy in medical writing (see Chapter 3). A computer program, described below, is available.

A little-known but very useful book is Neil Davis's *Medical Abbreviations: 24,000 Conveniences at the Expense of Communications and Safety*. All too often in medical writing, I encounter abbreviations for which I cannot find the explanation. Here are two randomly selected examples. What are the meanings of TDS and BEGA? Give up? TDS stands for traveler's diarrhea syndrome and BEGA stands for best estimate of gestational age. TEMP can mean temperature, temporary, or temporal. This little book can help clear up the confusion in ways I seldom could achieve looking in the indexes of my big reference books. I buy mine on line at www.medabbrev.com.

If you are taken with using classical medical quotations to augment your own prose, a good source is Maurice B. Strauss's *Familiar Medical Quotations* (Little, Brown). It is out of print, but is available from on-line booksellers: Do a Google search for Maurice Strauss AND medical quotations.

Computer Programs

Thesaurus
There is no need to buy a thesaurus. Your Microsoft Word program has an excellent one; just highlight the word and press shift/F7.

Electronic Medical Dictionary
I own *Stedman's Electronic Medical Dictionary* and keep it running whenever I am doing a writing task. Lippincott Williams & Wilkins reports that Version 6.0 "provides fast, easy access to over 104,000 fundamental and cutting-edge medical terms and features clearly written definitions, written and audio pronunciations, etymologies, images, tables, and anatomic animations." I don't really value the audio pronunciations (after all, I am writing—not giving a lecture) and spare me the anatomic animations. Also, I don't buy each new version published. That said, this is a very useful program to have loaded on your hard drive.

Spell Checker
I am a huge fan of *Stedman's Plus Medical/Pharmaceutical Spellchecker*. This amazing program integrates with your Microsoft Word spell checker. Then it works while you type to verify spellings of medical and pharmaceutical words plus the everyday words on the MS spell checker. The latest

version has the most recently released drug names, including brand names, and virtually all medical words you will ever use. It even has a feature that allows you to add words to its base. For example, *Dorland's* (the medical dictionary described above) was not in its vocabulary, so I added the word so that it will not be underlined in red next time I use it.

At this time, I should explain that I own no stock in Lippincott Williams & Wilkins Publishers. I do happen to be one of their authors, having published three books with them in the past. I am recommending so many of their products because I believe them to be the best available, undoubtedly because LWW has developed a focused line of books that are useful to all medical writers, including transcriptionists and medical secretaries. To find the series, go to www.lww.com and then to the key word "Stedman's."

Drug Reference Program
As an alternative or in addition to owning the *Quick Look Drug Book*, the *Quick Look Electric Drug Reference* (LWW, again) can be purchased and loaded on your hard drive.

Web Sites

Web sites are where the professionals look for information. In fact, the list of books and programs above may be unnecessary a decade from now. I am going to discuss my favorite sites; I think it is best to become really familiar with just a few and learn to use them well. This is much better than cruising a large number of sites but doing so inefficiently. Also, some of the best Web sites charge a subscription fee, which will put economic limits on your surfing. My medical school has subscriptions to MDConsult and UpToDate, as long as I access them from a university computer. However, I must pay a fee if I wish to use them at home. No matter which Web sites you choose as your personal favorites, you must learn to use them yourself. You cannot be dependent on the expertise of a medical librarian. And to be an effective Web searcher, you must understand Boolean searching.

Boolean Searching

Boolean logic, named for British-born Irish mathematician George Boole, refers to relationships between search terms. Fundamentally, it allows you and me to search the Web for the commonality, or maybe the lack thereof, of two possibly related items. It's not difficult. In a Boolean search, you will use one of three words to link two (or more) items. The words are AND, NOT, and OR. As an example, let's assume that I want to look up current information about the treatment of migraine headaches. I would first enter the terms migraine AND treatment. This will give me only articles about migraine therapy, and not information about the aura or the treatment of peptic ulcer disease. If I ask for migraine headache NOT treatment, I should get a list of articles about epidemiology, classification, symptoms, diagnosis, and so forth—all except therapy. And if I request migraine headache OR treatment, I should get it all.

Not clear yet? Let's try a metaphor: If I request yellow AND red, I should get orange. If I request yellow NOT red, I should get yellow only, and not green or even orange. If I request yellow OR red, I should get both red and yellow, and with some orange thrown in.

You can link more than two terms. The more terms you combine with AND, the shorter the list of articles created. The more terms linked with OR, the more articles on the list retrieved.

Many, but not all, Web sites allow Boolean searching.

Google

Don't laugh. Google, at http://www.google.com, is an outstanding search engine. If you want a quick link to a phrase, book title, author's name, or an unfamiliar Web site, try Google first. I have made it my Internet home page. The more you use Google the better you will like it. A second choice is http://www.dogpatch.com, but I like Google better.

If you have ever had an article published in an indexed journal, search your name on Google to see what you find. Or type in your home telephone number (all 10 digits, no punctuation), and then after seeing your street address appear, go to Yahoo! Maps to find a map to your home.

Google allows Boolean searching.

MEDLINE/PubMed

MEDLINE (Medical Literature, Analysis, and Retrieval System Online) is a service of the United States National Library of Medicine (NLM). It allows you to search up to 12 million references to life-science journal articles, chiefly those in the biomedical sciences. I prefer to search using PubMed, a service of the NLM that includes over 14 million citations from MEDLINE and other sources. Your search can go back to the 1950s.

You can access MEDLINE on the Internet by going to the NLM home page at http://www.nlm.nih.gov. There is no fee for use of this service and no requirement to register. You might also access MEDLINE through your medical library, public library, or a commercial Web site. An example of the latter is Physicians Online (http://www.pol.net), a Web site for physicians that offers e-mail service and current medical information, as well as MEDLINE/PubMed access. Registration for POL is required, but there is no charge. The easiest access is to go directly to PubMed via http://www.pubmed.com.

In PubMed you have choices: You can search by title word, phrase, text word, author name, journal name or any combination of these. PubMed allows Boolean searches. Your search will yield a list of citations to relevant journal articles, including the authors, title, publication source, and often an abstract. PubMed will search published scientific articles, but not books.

You can also search by using the NLM controlled vocabulary, MeSH. This abbreviation stands for Medical Subject Headings. MeSH is described as the NLM's controlled vocabulary thesaurus. The NLM fact sheet describes MeSH as follows: "It consists of sets of terms naming descriptors in a hierarchical structure that permits searching at various levels of specificity. MeSH descriptors are arranged in both an alphabetic and a hierarchical structure. At the most general level of the hierarchical structure are very broad headings such as 'Anatomy' or 'Mental Disorders.' At more narrow levels are found more specific headings such as 'Ankle' and 'Conduct Disorder.' There are 21,512 descriptors in MeSH."

Are you confused yet? I am. I have always considered MeSH headings to be the medical librarians' full employment act. I don't use it. If you really want to learn more, go to http://www.nlm.nih.gov/pubs/factsheets/mesh.html.

PubMed also offers "Loansome Doc," a feature that lets you place an electronic order for the full-text copy of an article found on MEDLINE/PubMed. The source is the National Network of Libraries of Medicine (NN/LM). You will need to register. You might also be able to link to the journal publisher's Web site and may be able to view a full text of an article. You may need to pay a fee.

MDConsult

MDConsult is a subscription-based (yes, this means a fee) Web site that allows you to access 40 medical reference books, more than 50 medical journals, and MEDLINE. It also contains an excellent reference base on some 30,000 medications, a number of clinical practice guidelines, and more than 3500 patient education handouts that can be customized. MDConsult allows Boolean searches. You can learn more about MDConsult at http://www.mdconsult.com.

I find MDConsult user-friendly and I like it. Its good point is that it combines medical reference book access with journals, and it has an excellent drug reference, with prices. When am working in the clinic with residents, I keep the Web site open and refer to it often.

UpToDate

I also like UpToDate, but for different reasons than I like MEDLINE/PubMed and MDConsult. UpToDate, also subscription based, is a clinical information source. What makes it different is that it offers state-of-the-art reviews of clinical subjects. The UpToDate Web site states, "Our topic reviews are written exclusively for UpToDate by physicians for physicians—nearly 3000 physicians serve as authors. Our content is comprehensive yet concise and it's fully referenced."

Of course this means that UpToDate is composed of "review articles," and is not really taking you to primary sources. Thus it is very useful for the busy clinician seeing patients, and I use it in teaching residents. UpToDate is designed to initially search a single subject, such as "headache." Then you will be offered a menu of modifiers such as: migraine, cluster, tension type, and so forth. You cannot do a Boolean search on UpToDate. For the medical writer, it is helpful to check current thinking on a topic. For primary sources of clinical evidence, I would look elsewhere. For further information about UpToDate, go to http://www.uptodate.com.

Uniform Requirements for Manuscripts Submitted to Biomedical Journals

The "Uniform Requirements" is a document approximately 31 pages long; one cannot search it. It is the Bible for the serious medical researcher, writer, and editor. I urge you to go to the Web site—http://www.icmje.org—and print a copy. You will use it often to answer questions, especially when writing reports of clinical research. What is it? *The Uniform Requirements for Manuscripts Submitted to Biomedical Journals*[9] tells medical writers how to prepare their manuscripts. Topics are listed in Table 1.3. The section Requirements for Submission of Manuscripts has excellent discussions of manuscript preparation, authorship, the various components of a research report (more on this in Chapter 9), and a section on how to cite references that you will find very valuable when working on your manuscripts.

Who writes the Uniform Requirements? The Uniform Requirements were first written in 1978, and first published in 1979. The initial authors were a small group of editors of general medical journals who met informally in Vancouver, British Columbia. This group has evolved into the International Committee of Medical Journal Editors (ICMJE). The group meets yearly, updates the document as needed, and has expanded its area of interest into the ethical issues and related concerns in medical publication, described as "Separate Statements."

TABLE 1.3. Topics covered in Uniform Requirements for Manuscripts Submitted to Biomedical Journals

Redundant or duplicate publication
Secondary publication
Protection of patients' right to privacy
Reporting guidelines for specific study designs
Requirements for submission of manuscripts
Sending the manuscript to the journal

TABLE 1.4.   Separate Statements Found in the Uniform Requirements for Manuscripts Submitted to Biomedical Journals

The definition of a peer-reviewed journal
Editorial freedom and integrity
Conflict of interest
Project-specific industry support for research
Corrections, retractions, and "expressions of concern" about research findings
Confidentiality
Medical journals and the popular media
Policies for posting biomedical journal information on the Internet
Advertising
Supplements
The role of the correspondence column
Competing manuscripts based on the same study
Differences in analysis or interpretation
Differences in reported methods or results

The topics in the section of "Separate Statements" are listed in Table 1.4. These are essentially policy statements written by the ICMJE. If one or more of these topics might be relevant to your paper, it would be a very good idea to review the statement.

WHERE DO I START IF I HAVE NEVER BEEN PUBLISHED?

The Medical Writer's Three Questions

In Puccini's opera *Turandot*, the Princess Turandot asks Prince Calef three questions, framed as riddles. If the love-struck prince answers the three queries correctly, he gets the princess's hand in marriage. If he fails, well, it's off with his head. For medical writers, also, there are three key questions that must be answered when considering a project: So what? Who cares? Where will my article be published?

For the medical writer—whether neophyte or seasoned—these questions are vital. If you answer the three questions clearly, you have the best chance of success. On the other hand, if you fail to provide a convincing answer to one or more of the questions, you won't exactly lose your head, but the success of your paper is definitely in jeopardy.

So What?

The medical landscape is littered with published papers that have accomplished little more than adding a few lines to the authors' curriculum vitae. If you aspire to add to the medical literature (or "*litter*-ature"), I urge you to be honest in considering the "So what?" question.

This question aims to determine the significance of your work. After all, undertaking a writing project is going to take you away from your patients, your family, yard work, cooking, travel, or whatever else you might be doing with your time. And you are asking your audience also to commit time to reading it. So be sure the effort is worthwhile.

The "So what?" questions asks: Is what I am writing about something that hasn't been said already, and perhaps said better than I will say it? Am I saying anything new? Let's assume that you are a surgeon writing for a surgical journal. If you are writing *The Surgical Treatment of Acute Appendicitis*, my first thought is that this topic may be important to me, but hasn't it already been said? But if your topic is *A New Surgical Technique for Appendectomy in the Patient with Acute Appendicitis*, then you have my attention.

Here is another example. One could study and report the diagnoses of the next 1000 patients seen in your office. But so what? On the other hand, if you studied the next 1000 patients seen with a presenting complaint of pelvic pain and followed them to the definitive diagnoses, then most generalists and gynecologists would be interested.

Who Cares?

This question has to do with relevance to the audience. A paper about a new appendectomy technique is not relevant to readers of a psychiatric journal. Okay, that is obvious. Let us think about a paper describing how I treat sore throats empirically with saline gargles and garlic, where I found that that the treated group actually fared significantly better than the control group. Although the topic seems unlikely, with good statistics this paper might be relevant to generalists who see many patients with sore throats.

When I was in private practice three decades ago, we often recommended that patients with peptic ulcer disease drink plenty of whole milk. Yes, things have changed. Nevertheless, it seemed that many patients with peptic ulcer disease reported not liking milk more often than expected. I thought of doing a study and writing it up. I asked my colleagues about this idea, and learned, to my dismay, that they really didn't care. I never did the study.

Where Will My Article be Published?
Getting an article published requires two consenting adults—an author and an editor. Of course, for refereed publications there are peer reviewers who must also nod approval. Even book publishers today have all proposals reviewed by experts in the field.

When you write an innovative, relevant article, you must seek the right audience. That means finding the best journal for your work. Ideally you begin with a specific publication in mind, your "target journal," and then drop back to your second and third choices only if you are not successful with your first choice.

Be careful with your target journal. Some journals have such a low acceptance rate that rejection is almost guaranteed. On the other end of the spectrum, the advertiser-sponsored publications (discussed below), while lacking the cachet of the *New England Journal of Medicine*, need a steady supply of innovative articles and offer good opportunities for the neophyte author. Some articles, by the nature of their content, are best suited for refereed journals that publish research reports; others—such as "how-to" and "five-ways-to" articles—are inappropriate for such journals and sending them in is a waste of time and postage.

Some Early Steps

Writing Models for Beginners
If you are a beginning author, it is difficult to write a report of original research on your first or second attempt. First, you need research data, which you are unlikely to have. Second, the report of original research is the most demanding of all publication models and holds the least chance of publication. There is one way in which this approach can work. That

occurs when you are the junior member of a research team, and you participate in all phases of the project, including writing the report. This approach works even better if the team includes a senior mentor, who can guide you through the process.

In the absence of a research team, research mentor, and pile of research data, what is the aspiring author to do? Plan to start with a writing model that offers the best chance of getting in print with the least need for expertise and the least effort. No, such a publication won't get you tenure or assure a lifelong career, but it will get you going. Also, it just might help you settle on a topic area that you can pursue in future writing.

The leading models appropriate for neophyte writers are review articles, case reports, editorials, letters, and book reviews. All are covered in depth in later chapters in the book. The review article is appealing because advertiser-supported publications, sometimes called "throw-aways," have a constant appetite for content. Examples of such publications are *Postgraduate Medicine*, *Consultant*, *The Female Patient*, *Hospital Practice*, and *Resident and Staff Physician*. All have Web sites for those who want to learn more.

Case reports are tempting, and are sometimes a good way to get started as a writer. Be sure of two things: One is that you have a point to make about the case—the "So what?" question again. The second is to be sure that your target journal(s) actually publishes case reports; not all journals do so. That is the "Where will my article be published?" question once more.

Editorials allow you to express opinions, and you may be an especially appropriate author for an editorial if you hold a position that gives you some expertise in the topic. For example, if you direct a pain clinic, you are qualified to write about narcotic abuse or underuse for patients with pain.

Letters to the editor are a quick and easy way to get in print. Generally a letter to the editor comments on a published paper. What you have to say must offer new insights and it must connect with the readers. Often such letters disagree with conclusions of the paper, and that is okay. Letters to the editor should be short and to the point.

Book reviews are another opportunity for publication. Never send in an unsolicited book review. On the other hand, you can write to your favorite journal and volunteer to be a book reviewer. If added to the reviewer list, you will receive a book to review. Your job will be to write the review, as described in Chapter 7. You keep the book as payment.

Book chapters are almost always invited, and book editors choose prospective authors from those writing on the topic needed for the book. You may be invited to write a book chapter after publishing a few articles on your new focus area, but book chapters are virtually never where a new writer begins. The same holds for writing a book. A few will succeed, but for most this is not where to start.

Mistakes We Make When Getting Started

- Trying to do it alone: If at all possible, work with someone more experienced. Your colleague may be a coauthor, or someone who reads your work and comments.
- Trying to run before you can walk: Do not attempt to write the definitive work on a topic or the grand epic in your specialty. Aim early to learn the writing and publication process by getting something written and in print, however humble your early pieces may seem. In my early days, I wrote for *Medical Economics* and *Physician's Management* on topics such as "Having Regular Meetings with Your Office Staff" and "How to See Patients More Efficiently in Your Office." I don't write on practice management subjects any more, but these articles helped me learn how to write and get published.
- Starting to write without preparation: It is a big mistake to begin writing until you have selected and refined your topic, figured out how you will structure your article, done your research, and assembled your writing tools. Without being prepared, inspiration won't carry you very far beyond page one. Starting off unprepared will almost surely lead to an uneven product, and you will spend a lot of time doing remedial work. It is much better to be ready when you start, and know where you are going.

The Value of Early Success

Do not underestimate the value of early success in medical writing. I urge you to strive for something in print early, for your own contribution to the 21st century time capsule. Seeing your work in print is an exciting affirmation of your self-worth. A few early publications will carry you through the effort of more writing and the rejections that are sure to come as you aim higher and higher. Also, try very hard to avoid a succession of early failures.

The next four chapters deal with basic writing skills that can help you win the publication race. The later chapters in the book describe the specific writing models, including "how-to" advice and problems to avoid. The last chapter has tips that can help you get your work published.

REFERENCES

1. Rew DA. Writing for readers. Eur J Surg Oncol 2003;29:633–634.
2. Batshaw ML, Plotnick LP, Petty BG, Woolf PK, Mellits ED. Academic promotion at a medical school: experience at Johns Hopkins University School of Medicine. N Engl J Med 1988;318:741–747.
3. Beasley BW, Wright SM. Looking forward to promotion: characteristics of participants in the Prospective Study of Promotion in Academia. J Gen Intern Med 2003;18:705–710.
4. Sebastian A. A dictionary of the history of medicine. New York: Parthenon; 1995.
5. Major RH. Classic descriptions of disease. Springfield, IL: Charles C Thomas; 1932.
6. Dirckx JH. The language of medicine. 2nd ed. New York: Praeger; 1983.
7. Porter R. A dictionary of the history of medicine. New York: Parthenon; 1999.
8. Hammer AL. Introduction to type and careers. Palo Alto, CA: Consulting Psychologists Press; 1995.
9. International Committee of Medical Journal Editors. Uniform requirements for manuscripts submitted to biomedical journals. Updated October 2001. http://www.icmje.org. Accessed November 2, 2003.

2
Basic Writing Skills

Do not skip this chapter. Yes, there will be the temptation to go directly to the chapter describing the article you want to write, but that would be a mistake. It would be like attempting to build a house without a blueprint and tools. In writing an article or a book chapter, the topic is what you want to "build." The structure is your blueprint, and the paragraphs, sentences, and words are the contents of your toolbox. So learn your craft and how to use your tools before starting to construct your masterpiece.

Much of this chapter is fundamental English 101—just adapted to medical writing. However, it is not a comprehensive course in English composition and grammar. In fact, if my English teachers from high school and college ever read this they might say, "Bob, is this all you remember of what I taught you?" It is not really all I recall, but it represents the Cliff Notes—the bare bones of what the medical writer needs to know.

IDEA DEVELOPMENT

The Great Idea

A good idea is the most important thing a medical writer can have. It can come to you in a variety of ways. One might be as a result of a discussion with colleagues, as happened to me a few years ago. At that time, there had been a sudden drop in students matching in my specialty. Yet, in trying to place an unmatched student in a residency program using phone contacts, I encountered inefficiency and almost indifference— all from residency directors who had vacancies and whom I assumed really needed to recruit students into their programs. I described this phenomenon at our department's weekly faculty meeting and reported briefly what I thought the residency directors needed to know. In my remarks to the faculty, I listed five things that residency directors should do to be receptive to unmatched students attempting to "scramble." And then I thought: Why not write it up? I returned to my office and finished the short piece by noon. It was published a few months later.[1]

A second source of ideas should be your area of interest and expertise. For example, I was recently asked by a medical journal to write an editorial; almost any topic would be okay. I considered the significance of a current whooping cough scare, the health risks to travelers in the holiday season, and even the changing demographics of medical school classes. In the end, I decided to do what I should do, and that is to write about what I know. I did some research and wrote a nice, short editorial, "How Physicians Read the Medical Literature."[2] The journal editor liked the topic and how I handled it, and no readers wrote to say that I was misguided or uninformed. Also, some of what I learned was useful in planning Chapter 5 of this book.

A third possibility is looking at clinical implications of current public issues. Here is an example: From time to time, I teach a course in medical writing for faculty members at our medical school. This course involves 90-minute sessions held once a month over 6 or 8 months. The course is for beginning medical writers, and one objective is to have each participant write a review paper and have it on its way into publication before the last session ends. In our current course, one faculty member with a certificate of added qualifications in geriatrics plans to write "Assessing Older Persons for Their Ability to Operate a Motor Vehicle Safely." She has a very good idea, timely and clinically relevant. (I will discuss below how she developed the idea.) As a course assignment, she called a review journal editor to discuss the article; the response was very positive, with a discussion of holding a spot for the article in a future issue. By the time this book is published, the article will probably be in print.

The points I have tried to make in the anecdotes above are:

■ When something excites you and you have, you believe, an answer to a current problem (such as residency directors needing to learn to "scramble"), think about writing it up. Then do it now, before the idea gets cold.

■ Write on what you know about and what interests you. This helps maintain your interest and also helps focus your writing on the topic that will move your career along.

■ Write on clinical topics in your area of expertise. In general, medical publications need articles about practical aspects of disease diagnosis and management. And, of course, research journals need reports of original research studies.

Allowing the Idea to Incubate

Generally you should let your idea germinate for a while. I recognize that I am mixing my metaphors, but I like to think of this activity as "free-range" accumulation of odd facts, phrases, and connections. Thoughts will come into your head in the shower or while driving your car. Sometimes they occur in the middle of a meeting, when a comment creates a synapse in the writing center of your brain. Ideas about your writing may appear in that shadow land between wakefulness and REM (rapid eye movement) sleep. Do not lose these thoughts! You have been blessed with a gift that may make your article better. Write it down. Enter it in your portable computer. Put it in your journal. Scribble it on an old envelope. Whatever you do, hang on to it, and don't let it get away. Many times I have left a shower or a warm bed to jot down a writing idea that I knew would escape if not captured at that moment.

For example, the metaphor of the "free-range" accumulation of items to flesh out an idea occurred to me during a long airplane ride; it was Thanksgiving time and I had read about "free-range" turkeys that sought their food in a more or less natural way. Not being one who carries a computer when traveling, I jotted the phrase on the blank sheet of paper I always carry for this purpose. Now here it is in print, courtesy of United Airlines and foolscap, and then my notebook computer. It may not be the brightest idea I ever had, but at least it didn't get away. A better example may be the analogy, described in Chapter 1, of the three questions asked by Princess Turandot of the prince and the three questions writers must answer about their current work; this occurred to me while listening to a very long aria from Puccini's opera, and I jotted the idea on the printed program.

In preparing to write this book, I created a file that lists each chapter. Under each chapter I record miscellaneous notes, brilliant thoughts, literary allusions, and short paragraphs that seem witty. Then I go to this "Notes" file as I begin to write each chapter.

Focusing the Topic

Most article ideas we get are too broad, and an early task is generally to limit the focus. Here is an example: Let's say that I want to write an article about the diagnosis of headache. This topic is much too broad, and so I might limit it first by focusing on the diagnosis of a type of headache, such as migraine, tension type, or even cluster headache. But these topics are still too broad. Let's choose migraine headache, and limit it some more. We might discuss diagnosis of migraine headache in women, in children, or in the elderly; the implications are clinically different in each. Another way to approach the diagnosis of migraine is to consider when diagnostic imaging (computed tomography or magnetic resonance imaging) is needed. Now we are getting more specific. In the end, a good topic and title might be: "When is Diagnostic Imaging Needed in the Diagnosis of Childhood Headache?" Or another approach could be: "Red Flags in the Headache History: Five Reasons to Obtain Diagnostic Imaging."

The astute writer avoids telling too much. This helps prevent "overwriting"—producing an article much too long for any journal and thus in need of ruthless pruning. By this I mean that if your article is about when to seek diagnostic imaging in a headache patient, you should make it clear to your reader (and to yourself) that you will not discuss what blood tests to order, drugs and doses, or special diets. You will plan ahead and stick to your topic.

Jotting notes and focusing the topic help move you to the next step—planning the concept and structure of your article.

ARTICLE STRUCTURE

Your article or chapter is intended to provide information or answer questions for your readers. To achieve this goal, you must present your information in the best possible format. Possibilities include the review article, editorial, case report, letter to the editor, book chapter, or report of original research. Each has its own rules for structure, and will be covered in chapters to come. At this time, I will use the review article format to discuss article structure. I choose this format since the review article allows the writer the greatest opportunity to express creativity in how to handle material.

Sometimes the focused topic yields the concept. In the instance of "Red Flags in the Headache History: Five Reasons to Obtain Diagnostic Imaging," the article structure is self-evident: The article will begin with an introduction stating the epidemiology and background for the problem. Next will come a five-part section on the red flags, which would include migraine associated with a neurologic abnormality on physical examination (such as unexplained unilateral deafness or weakness in an extremity), a seizure, or a trajectory of increasing pain and frequency of headaches. Last will come the summary/discussion section that pulls it all together. With this structure, the article practically writes itself.

The secret of structuring an article is finding the topic's component parts. An article on treating back pain may have four components: medications, physical therapy, determination of appropriate activity levels, and preventing future recurrences. If writing a piece on diagnosing depression in teenagers, I might cover what teens face in life each day, symptoms of depression that teens may exhibit, and how to confirm a diagnostic hunch. I might even include a table, "High Pay-Off Questions to Help Spot the Depressed Teenager." Such a table might prove especially useful to readers.

In the end, the focused topic and presentation concept should evolve into an outline. Yes, an outline. Your feelings about a high school English teacher might have turned you against outlines, but they are usually an important key to writing success. In planning this book, I developed a 12-page expanded outline that gave the topics for each chapter down to the third level of topic heading. Of course, as I write each chapter, I may rearrange things a little, but the overall outline tells me where I am going and what will be presented in each chapter and under which heading. It also, I hope, helps me avoid too much repetition.

In planning the article cited above on assessing driving skills in the elderly, our faculty member decided on the following preliminary outline:

Introduction
    Background, including statistics
    Legal aspects of the problem
Areas to assess
    Mental competence and dementia
    Physical competence and handicaps
    Special senses
      Vision
      Hearing
    Medications
Making decisions
    Dealing with the patient
    State laws
    Family issues
Conclusion

In general there are some time-tested ways to structure articles. Of course, if you are writing a report of original research, you must, repeat *must*, use the IMRAD model, which describes Introduction, Methods, Results, and Discussion; this will be described in detail in Chapter 9. If writing a book chapter or review article on a disease such as gastroesophageal reflux disease (GERD), the headings are likely to be Background, Clinical History, Physical Examination, Laboratory Tests and Imaging, Treatment Options, and Prevention.

For other articles, general approaches might be:

The List

This is my favorite way to organize a review article or an editorial. Examples might be:

Three exercises that may prevent back pain
Four herbal remedies for chronic joint pain
Five ways to improve collections in your office practice
Six questions that can help diagnose panic disorder.

What's New?

A new procedure for ventral hernia repair

A new federal regulation that will affect your practice

A review of new treatment regimens for AIDS

New drugs to treat fungal infections of the skin.

Questions and Answers

What are safe antibiotics to use in pregnancy?

Who should perform head and neck surgery?

What vaccines should be given to the international traveler?

What are the early signs of pancreatic cancer?

Current Controversies

Dementia and the statins: Do the drugs prevent or cause dementia?

Who should or should not receive flu shots?

Who should receive outpatient laparoscopic cholecystectomy?

The ethical issues in boutique medical practice.

Mistakes We Make in Article Structure

Beginning writers often make the following mistakes in defining the concept and structure of their articles:

- Starting to write without a concept. Having a good idea is wonderful, but you must also decide how you will handle the idea.
- Attempting to write without an outline. Maybe some creative and experienced writers can do so, but for the beginning medical writer, an outline is a must. As I compose this chapter today, my outline is located to my left on my desk.
- Having an outline with too many major headings and not enough development of each. More than five main headings in the outline is almost certainly too many for a medical article. Please notice that this chapter, which is about

twice the length of a medical article, has only five main headings.

■ Trying to cover too much ground. Focus, limit, and then narrow some more.

■ Failing to introduce the purpose of the article very early in the writing.

■ Developing a good concept and structure, and then failing to follow the blueprint. Editors will quickly spot when you have left the main highway and strayed off on a side path.

■ Beginning to write the manuscript without thinking the project through. This will only lead to much painful rewriting later. Clear writing comes from clear thinking. See the completed project in your mind before starting the first paragraph.

PARAGRAPH DEVELOPMENT

A paragraph is a collection of sentences that all relate to a common theme. In a sense, each paragraph is a small essay. This means that you should follow the basic rules for writing an essay: tell your reader what you are trying to say early in the essay, develop the theme using some concrete examples, then conclude in a thoughtful way. In an essay, sometimes it is good to reprise the opening sentence in some way, and this can also work well in a paragraph. An alternative conclusion to a paragraph may be a transition to the next paragraph. Choose your ending, and then move on.

The first sentence in a paragraph is classically the "topic sentence." The topic sentence states what the paragraph is about and is thus probably going to be somewhat general in nature. Let's look at the paragraph just before this one: The topic sentence is "A paragraph is a collection of sentences that all relate to a common theme." Then the paragraph goes on to give three steps in developing the paragraph: (1) state the topic early; (2) use examples; and (3) conclude in a meaningful way, perhaps with a hint of transition to the next topic. This is classic paragraph development.

There are occasional exceptions to the classic format, such as when the example is stated first to get the reader's attention, followed by the general statement telling what the example means. Here is a demonstration of what I mean:

Over-the-counter drug availability and unintended consequences
  Initial example to get the reader's attention:

  > Since H2-blockers became available over the counter (OTC) in drugstores, physicians have reported that some public assistance patients have ceased their use of these medications and are experiencing recurrences of epigastric distress.

  General statement relating the significance of the example:

  > Sometimes regulations that are intended to make drugs more available to patients have a paradoxical effect of reducing their use. [The paragraph will go on to explain why— because welfare patients could previously get the H2-blocker drugs at no personal cost by prescription, but now that the drugs are available OTC, they are no longer eligible for prescription coverage and patients must pay for the medication.]

Organizing the Paragraph

Thoughts in a paragraph must be presented in an orderly fashion, not jumbled like a bag of toys. Sentences can be arranged in a chronology of what happens. I used this in the preceding paragraphs: moving from topic sentence, to examples, to conclusion. Or you may decide to order sentences by rank of importance. In describing causes of a low back pain, you might mention lumbosacral strain (the most common cause) first, then herniated lumbar disc (less common, but very important), followed by less common causes such as spinal abscess, metastatic cancer, and so forth. An alternative method of ordering sentences within a paragraph might be a reverse ranking order: In this setting you might describe the medications currently used to treat peptic ulcer disease, briefly describing the least expensive or the least effective ones first, and then spending most of the space on today's popular remedy, the protein pump inhibitors. Or sometimes the rational order is nothing more than a simple list. In this paragraph I told you about four ways to organize sentences in a paragraph, presented in no particular order.

When you have finished writing a paper, try this test to see whether you have organized your paragraphs well. Begin with a paper copy of your manuscript and some colored highlight markers. Then first highlight in yellow (or another favorite color) the key sentence in each paragraph; the sentences highlighted in yellow should, in most instances, be at the beginning of each paragraph.

Next, use another color (let's say blue) to highlight the examples that support the key general statement. Most or all paragraphs should have supporting facts, and they should generally follow the yellow-highlighted topic sentence. The exception, as noted above, will be when the example is used as the lead item in the paragraph. In the next section, we will spend some more time considering supporting examples.

Using Concrete Examples

At times you will read a paper and think, This is dull. When this happens, ask yourself why. Often the answer is that the writer has written in broad general statements, and failed to provide examples to illustrate theory. This happens especially in philosophy and sometimes in the psychological literature. Medical writers are often spared this transgression because we present specific data such as laboratory tests, drugs, and doses. Nevertheless, we must be vigilant about unsupported general assertions.

Why do we see writing without examples? Here is one reason: Writing general statements is easy. We all like to share our great ideas. But thinking up examples to support our favorite philosophical thoughts is often a struggle. Finding specific examples can be difficult, but concrete facts are what make writing come alive.

To illustrate the use of examples to clarify general statements, let us look at three examples:

■ *Role of the primary care physician*
General statement:

> The primary care physician must be the expert in the care of common illnesses and in the recognition of uncommon diseases.

Example:

> The general internist or family physician should be skilled in the management of degenerative joint disease, and able to differentiate it from rheumatoid arthritis, intraarticular infection, and other causes of joint pain.

■ *Changing our minds about the use of drugs*
General statement:

> Sometimes we find that drugs once avoided in certain diseases actually can be helpful.

Example:

> It was once axiomatic that one did not prescribe beta-blocker drugs for patients with congestive heart failure, but now we have discovered that the drugs are useful in treating some heart failure patients.

■ *Use of influenza vaccine in early pregnancy*
General statement:

> In this age of evidence-based medicine, some recommendations seem to be based on intuition or tradition, rather than the results of scientific studies.

Example:

> Influenza vaccine is generally not given during the first trimester of pregnancy, although there are no published controlled studies to support this practice.

Being Considerate of Your Reader

Be considerate of your reader by making your paragraphs not too long, not too short, and not too dense. In medical writing, paragraphs often seem to go on for pages and pages; that may be a little exaggerated, but when the prose is unnecessarily burdened with long medical words and phrases, and when there is sentence after sentence without a break, the resulting paragraph becomes just too long. Whenever you find a paragraph that continues for more than eight or 10 sentences, look and see whether there is a logical break in the middle, even if you need to add a transition phrase or sentence. If a paragraph covers two or more topics, it almost certainly needs to be divided into two.

Don't make your paragraphs too short. I generally like short paragraphs. They allow more pleasing "white space" on the page, and they give the reader time to breathe. That said, we must remember that a paragraph is, as noted above, a collection of sentences that relate to a common topic. One or two silver dollars do not make a collection, and most paragraphs need more than one or two sentences. Are there exceptions? Yes, the exception is when a one-sentence paragraph is used for emphasis. But, like a person who sends e-mail messages laden with exclamation points or shouts while talking, using more than the occasional one-sentence paragraph will irritate the reader.

How you construct your paragraphs affects the density of the page. We like journals and books in part because of the information contained and part because of their pleasant appearance. The computer screen has not yet equaled the pleasure of holding and reading something with printed pages. Part of the pleasure of the printed page is what is *not* there. By that I mean, there must be a balance of printed word and, as mentioned briefly above, "white space"—the area of the page that has no ink. On any page there is probably an amount of white space that is just right. This is achieved by alternating paragraph length, avoiding an article with all very long paragraphs (tiresome) or all very short paragraphs (annoying), and perhaps by using tables or figures (discussed in Chapter 4).

The density of the printed page is also managed by the use of headings. I have made liberal use of headings in this book. This allows the presentation of white space to frame the paragraphs, and does so in a way that I hope you find aesthetically appealing. After all, the pleasant appearance of the pages is part of the joy of reading.

SENTENCES

Active Versus Passive Voice

Here is a single answer quiz. Which is better? Pick one.

1. We found that ...
2. It was found that ...

About two decades ago, several colleagues and I submitted a paper to a prestigious academic journal. It described an innovative medical school clerkship for students. Our paper read something like this: "We identified a need in the curriculum. We developed and presented a six-week clerkship for the students. At the end of the year, we evaluated the outcome of the endeavor." Following appropriate peer review, the journal editor wrote to us, accepting the paper contingent on certain modifications. One of these modifications was that we authors change all statements to passive voice. And so, we laboriously revised our prose to read: "A need was identified for an addition to the curriculum. A clerkship was developed and presented. The outcomes were evaluated at the end of the year." In due time, the paper was published, but what was presented in print lacked the punch of what we originally submitted, and actually took more words to express the same thoughts.

If active voice has more vigor than passive, why do we use the latter? Somehow, it may seem easier to express our thoughts in passive voice, and perhaps we thereby take a little less responsibility for them when "I" or "we" is not stated. I wonder if we are more likely to use active voice when we feel confident about positive results in research and passive voice when our confidence is lacking or the results are equivocal. Another theory is proposed by Day[3]: "Perhaps this bad habit [using passive voice] is the result of the erroneous idea that it somehow impolite to use first-person pronouns."

We are definitely moving toward using more active voice in medical writing, especially in reporting original research. Here are some representative phrases from medical journals that have crossed my desk recently:

From *The Lancet* (2004;363:112–118):
  "We followed up children once a day for diarrhoea and a month for anthropometry…"
From the *New England Journal of Medicine* (2004; 350:114–124):
  "We enrolled 518 patient with polycythemia vera, …"

From the *British Medical Journal* (2001;323:382–386):
"I searched the Cochrane Library, Medline, and Embase to
identify studies of common pathological findings in..."

There are, of course, times when the use of passive voice is
best. The classical example is when who does something is less
important than the recipient of the action. In this instance it
may be better to say that "the patient was injected with the test
drug" rather than "we injected the test drug into the patient."
Or perhaps it doesn't matter who performed the action, just
that it occurred. For example, in the statement "The patient
was transported to the hospital by ambulance," it does not
matter who drove the vehicle.

Construct Sentences with Care

Words per Sentence

We medical writers often write jumbled and tortuous sentences. We try to put too much into them and we forget that
the best sentences contain one thought. When a sentence is
too long it may become barely intelligible. As an example of an
unfriendly sentence, I am going to rewrite the last paragraph
on page 40. Here goes:

> The density of the printed page is managed by how we use
> headings, and you will note that I have made liberal use of
> headings in the book, which allows the presentation of white
> space to frame my usually well-written paragraphs, doing so
> in a way that is aesthetically pleasing, which is, after all, part
> of the joy of reading a book.

This 63-word stinker of a sentence did not even trigger my
Microsoft Word grammar and spell checker to tell me that it
is too long—but it is, even with the relatively small words it
contains. Imagine how bad it could be if weighed down with
long scientific words or unfamiliar abbreviations.

If you have more than about 25 or 30 words or more than
two commas in a sentence, consider breaking it into two sentences, and you will usually find that it will read better. As an
example, I wrote the previous sentence—on purpose—using

34 words and combining two thoughts. Now let's rewrite it as two sentences:

> If you have more than about 25 or 30 words in a sentence, consider breaking it into two sentences. You will usually find that it will read better.

Do you agree that the rewrite is an improvement?

Words per Verb

If a sentence seems weak, count the words per verb. Verbs, the action words, are your strong words in a sentence. More than 20 words per verb tend to create a weak sentence. Here are the thoughts in the previous three sentences, considerably rewritten into one with 37 words and only one verb ("makes"):

> The use of an excessive number of words in conjunction with a single verb makes for a weak sentence, deficient in strong words, often complex in structure, and very likely complicated by a number of subordinate clauses.

Using Variety in Your Sentences

To make your writing vibrant, be sure to vary your sentence beginnings, type, and length.

Try to avoid using the same word repeatedly, especially at the beginning of the sentence. Also, try to have some simple declarative sentences, some a little complex, and some that even begin with prepositional phrases.

We have already discussed excessive sentence length, which can be tiresome to the reader. On the other hand, using too many short sentences is also poor writing.

The following is intended to illustrate all three points—sentence beginnings, type, and length:

> The elderly patient fell on a scatter rug at home. The patient struck his shoulder when he landed. The patient sustained a fracture of left humerus.

The three sentences all begin alike, are all simple and declarative, and are all quite short. No one of the sentences is improper in any way, but taken together, the writing is unskill-ful. A much better way to express the three facts would be:

> The elderly patient fell on a scatter rug at home, striking his shoulder and sustaining a fracture of the left humerus.

Sentence Density

Single sentences, like paragraphs, can be too dense for com-prehension by mere mortals. Consider the following sentence from a recent report with the very clear title "Effect of Improving Depression Care on Pain and Functional Out-comes Among Older Adults with Arthritis." This is a topic of interest to all of us who treat elderly patients. And so I read with great interest the first of two sentences in the Results section of the Abstract:

> In addition to reduction in depressive symptoms, the intervention group compared with the usual care group at 12 months had lower mean (SE) scores for pain intensity (5.63 [0.16] vs. 6.15 [0.16]; between-group difference, −0.53; 95% confidence interval (CI), −0.92 to −0.14; P = .009), interference with daily activities due to arthritis (4.40 [0.18] vs. 4.99 [0.17]; between-group difference, −0.59; 95% CI, −1.00 to −0.19; P = .004), and interference with daily activities due to pain (2.92 [0.07] vs. 3.17 [0.07]; between-group difference, −0.26; 95% CI, −0.41 to −0.10; P = .002).
> (*Source: JAMA 2003;290:2428.*)

As a practicing physician and a medical writer, what are my issues with this sentence and how could it have been improved? First, it is much too long and convoluted. I believe that it could have been divided into three or four shorter sen-tences to enhance clarity. Second, the abbreviation CI (for confidence interval) is explained, but SE remains a mystery and is not explained elsewhere in the Abstract. Finally, the sentence is, in my opinion, much too stuffed with data. Do I really need all of these numbers in the abstract? What has been saved for the Results section of the article?

Fortunately, the authors translate the difficult sentence for us mere mortals, and do so in very clear English: "In a large and diverse population of older adults with arthritis (mostly osteoarthritis) and comorbid depression, benefits of improved depression care extended beyond reduced depressive symptoms and included decreased pain as well as improved functional status and quality of life." Okay, even this sentence is a little long and complicated, but I can read it without difficulty. And I like that the author used simple words such as "mostly" instead of "predominantly" and "osteoarthritis" rather than "degenerative joint disease." I will present more on words in the next section.

Cadence
Sentences have a cadence that the reader can sense, much like the rhythm in a song. You can best sense the cadence by reading the sentence aloud. If a sentence is convoluted by too many clauses or if it is weighed down by too many unnecessary long words, the pleasant rhythm is lost. For example, take the first sentence in this paragraph, beginning, "Sentences have a cadence..." It's not Haiku poetry, but I think the sentence has a nice rhythm. It has several short words, then a long word, and no words with more than two syllables. Could the sentence be worse? Yes, it could. Here's how:

> Very analogous to the rhythm that may be found in a song, we are readily able to discern cadences that are found in sentences when they are well constructed.

Ugh! The sentence is syntactically correct, but not pleasing to read. Make your reading a pleasure for the reader, if you can. If you wonder about the cadence of your sentences, read them aloud.

Punctuation: Commas, Periods, and More

Commas, semicolons, periods, and question marks are called stops. They improve sentence cadence and clarity, and thus make reading easier. According to Jordan and Shepard,[4] "the stops should fit with the rhythm of respiration as well as with the sense of what is said."

Commas

Commas, like all stops, serve to break up the flow of words. Consider the sentence just before this one, and how it would read without commas:

> Commas like all stops serve to break up the flow of words.

I suspect that you would need to read it twice to discern my meaning, and then would mentally insert the commas.

The placement of commas can actually change meaning. For example:

> The physician thought the patient looked gravely ill.

Or

> The physician, thought the patient, looked gravely ill.

The presence or absence of commas changes who seemed ill.

Bernstein[5] has reported how the state of Michigan discovered that its state constitution inadvertently legalized slavery. Section 8, Article 2 read:

> Neither slavery nor involuntary servitude, unless for the punishment of a crime, shall ever be tolerated in this state.

Upon consideration, it was decided to delete the comma after servitude and place it after slavery.

Semicolons

The semicolon is used when you almost need a period; yet, a period would break up linked thoughts. If I used a period to divide the previous sentence, I would have created two short sentences in sequence. It might be acceptable, but joining the two thoughts with a semicolon seems right to me. In the setting of related thoughts and phrases, the use of semicolons is often a matter of individual style.

Semicolons are very useful in a series of items when the comma is needed within items. For example:

> Musculoskeletal injuries may be treated with rest; analgesics or muscle relaxant medication; and physical therapy including heat, ice, and stretching exercises.

Periods and Question Marks

The period is the "full stop" that ends a sentence. Period. Oh, yes, there are some technical uses, such as in abbreviations (e.g., Mr., Ph.D., or Dr.), but these do not affect sentence flow.

The question mark is an interrogatory symbol that appears after a direct question. A period is used with an indirect question. For example:

■ The direct question:

> The physician asked the patient, "Where is the pain located?"

■ The indirect question:

> The physician asked the patient where the pain was located.

Sentences with Misplaced Phrases

Do you remember the old song titled, "Throw Momma from the Train a Kiss?" Jumbled sentences with goofy phrases can find their way into the medical literature. The classic "Throw Momma..." sentence mixes up phrases within the sentence, together with a single verb that could apply to either phrase— albeit with potentially hazardous consequences in one of the two possibilities. In this example, the object of the verb "kiss" should follow the verb "throw" directly, with the less important prepositional phrase "from the train" relegated to the end of the sentence. Rewriting the sentence then gives us:

> Throw momma a kiss from the train.

Sentences with Verbose Phrases

Verbosity is a disease that afflicts many sentences in medical writing. Verbosity is simply using a long phrase to express a thought when fewer words will do nicely. A classical example is saying "fewer in number" instead of "less" or even "fewer." Or a careless author might write, "has the capability to" when meaning to say "can."

Table 2.1 presents a list of verbose phrases.

TABLE 2.1.   Verbose phrases: Why use one word when more will do?

Verbose phrase	What you mean to say
At this time	Now
At the conclusion of	After
With the exception of	Except
In only a small number of cases	Rarely
In many instances	Often
In light of the fact that	Because
More often than not	Usually
In the absence of	Without
On a daily basis	Daily
In close proximity to	Near
The great majority of	Most
With regard to	About
In the event that	If
In the not too distant future	Soon
Consensus of opinion	Consensus

Of course, it is not just phrases that are afflicted with wordiness. Sometimes entire sentences are involved. Here is one:

> The thesis is herein offered that woman (like man) is a biological, social and cultural creature, and as such is dependent for health on the acceptance, approval, support, and encouragement of significant individual members of the social group to which she belongs.

What the author means to say, I believe, is that a woman's health can be influenced by her peer relationships.

You can usually spot a verbose sentence before you are halfway through. How? Because it often begins with a phrase like:

- We are reminded of the necessity for the consideration of . . .
- Although certainly not a new finding, it is pertinent to remind the reader that . . .
- At this time, it be emphasized that . . .
- It is a well-recognized fact that . . .
- Let me make clear that . . .
- It is interesting to note that . . .

Of course, all this verbosity is really an excess of words, and often large words. So let's next consider our most basic tools—words.

WORDS

Words are the most basic tools we use to write. Winston Churchill once wrote: "Short words are best and old words, when short, are best of all." Sir Winston's sentence has a pleasing cadence. It uses the active voice. It is not long and convoluted. Most important, it uses only short words; in fact, the sentence contains only words of one syllable. They are old-fashioned English-language words, even though, like most words, they can be traced to some language in antiquity. Also, the sentence does not contain the complex scientific words we often must use in medical writing. One of the inescapable difficulties in medical writing is our dependence on scientific words derived from the classical languages. Their specificity is a benefit, but their complexity can become a curse in medical writing. Let's look at a few medical words.

Understanding Medical Words

I have always been fascinated by medical words, and I try hard to know the origins of those I use. I advise medical students and residents to keep a "medical word journal" to help them learn the classical roots, and various other origins, of words we use in clinical care. I believe that knowing the etymologic derivation of words such as *acetabulum* (from the Greek word for "vinegar cup") and *Norwalk virus* (from the small town in Ohio where the microorganism was first isolated) might make me a better writer. Even if this theory is flawed, knowing how these words arose enriches my life.

Most medical words come from Latin and Latinized Greek. The Latinization of Greek began when the Romans conquered the Greeks, and they appropriated everything, including their language. Later, in the post-Renaissance era, scholars and scientists turned to these languages as new words were needed to describe their discoveries. Also, as theorized by Dirckx[6]: "But there was a second and no less cogent reason: Latin was a dead language. No longer anyone's mother tongue, it was hardly more subject to alteration or corruption through use than the alphabet or multiplication table." Examples of words coming from Latin and Latinized Greek are *dementia* (to be mad), *placenta* (a flat cake), *gingiva* (gum), *scabies* (to scratch), *rubella* (diminutive of red), and *digitalis* (from digit, meaning finger or toe, and used because the drug came from foxglove, also called "ladies' fingers").

Later, the Anglo-Saxon tongues gave us *sick*, *blood*, and *gut*. (The latter is now the name of a prestigious journal.) Middle English gave us some medical words such as *eye* and Italian contributed *belladonna* (meaning beautiful lady). Others that are borrowed from foreign languages include *beriberi* (from the Singhalese word *beri* meaning weak; the doubling indicates extreme weakness) and *ammonia* from the Egyptian word for Jupiter (the rest of the story is that Jupiter was called Jupiter Ammon, and many persons came riding camels to worship the god at the shrine near the Libyan city of Ammonia; from the accumulated camel dung came a substance that was named ammonia). *Bezoar* came from a Persian word meaning antidote, and *quinine* arose from the Spanish spelling of the Peruvian word *kina*, meaning bark (of a tree).

Some medical words come from literature or mythology. These include *pickwickian syndrome*, *panic*, *syphilis*, *atlas*, *Munchausen syndrome*, and *Achilles tendon*. Some more recent medical neologisms involve places: the disease name *tularemia* comes from Tulare county in California, where the disease was first described. Even universities and patients get in the game: Warfarin, first marketed as a rat poison, is named after the *W*isconsin *A*lumni *R*esearch *F*oundation plus the last four letters of its chemical name; and the name *bacitracin* comes from "baci" for bacteria and "tracin" for Margaret Tracey, whose wound drainage permitted identification of the antibiotic.

Table 2.2 lists some of my favorite medical words and their origins. I hope that this section and the table inspire you to seek the sources, as well as the definitions, of unfamiliar words as you encounter them.

TABLE 2.2. The origins of selected medical words

Medical word	Origin of the word
Botulism	From German *botulismus*, meaning "sausage." In the Victorian times and later, Germans contracted the disease by eating sausage.
Carotid	From Greek *karotikos*, meaning "to render unconscious." The ancient Greeks noted what happened when you compressed these arteries.
Clap	Although not a proper medical term, the word comes from medieval French word *clapier*, meaning "brothel."
Hysteria	In ancient Greek the word *hustera* ("womb") evolved to *husterikos* ("malfunctioning womb"). I will say no more about this.
Influenza	Our word for flu borrowed the Italian word *influenza*, meaning "influence." They believed the disease was due to the power of the heavens.
Mastoid	From Greek *mastos*, meaning "breast." This is the shape of the postauricular bony outcropping of the temporal bone.
Mitral	The valve looks like a bishop's miter, his official headdress. Both come from the Greek word *mitra*, describing a cloth headband or girdle.
Penis	The word *penis* in Latin originally meant "tail."
Quarantine	From Latin *quadraginta*, meaning "forty." In medieval Venice and other ports, vessels were moored offshore for 40 days before being allowed to enter the port. This time exceeded the incubation period of most infectious diseases.
Thalassemia	From Greek *thalassa*, meaning "sea," and *haima*, the word for blood. The disease affected chiefly those who lived near the Mediterranean Sea.
Tsutsugamushi (fever)	This is the Japanese word meaning "dangerous bug."
Vitamin	When it was noted that an amine of nicotinic acid prevented pellagra, it was called a "vital amine," shortened to "vitamine" by a biochemist with the euphonious name Casimir Funk. Use of the word was expanded to include other compounds, some not actually amines, and hence the final "e" was eliminated.

Some Thoughts About the Types of Words We Use

We use many types of words, which include nouns and pronouns, verbs, modifiers such as adjectives and adverbs, metaphors and similes, onomatopoeic words and alliteration, literary allusions and eponyms.

Nouns and Pronouns

Nouns are persons and things: *doctor, disease, cat, dog, house.* They are generally strong words and classically occur early in a sentence. For example: The noun occurs first in the simple sentence, "The physician treated the patient." Short nouns make for easier reading than longer ones, but, as noted, this is sometimes not possible in medical writing, as we sacrifice readability to precision. We seldom get in trouble with nouns.

Pronouns are another story. We sometimes confuse pronouns and their antecedents—the word the pronoun replaces, as in the following:

> A new vaccine is available to prevent the flu, and to get it you should see your doctor now.

> This disease stands unique as the first truly American disease, and the guiding spirit that made this accomplishment possible is..."

> The resident anesthetized the patient as the attending surgeon waited; he then made the incision in the abdomen.

Over the past few years we have discovered another way to introduce complexity with pronouns, namely the use of clumsy neologisms to avoid the perception of sexist language. Newly created unisex pronouns have included "shim" and "s/he." Or, in the quest for gender-neutral writing, we have also begun to accept constructions such as, "The physician should treat their patient with respect." Probably the best of the compromises is the use of plural pronouns ("they") or using both genders ("he or she," "her or him"). In this book you will not find "their" used with a single noun as an antecedent. I have tried to minimize the use of wordy phrases such as "he or she" or "him or her," but found that I could not avoid their use altogether.

Verbs

Verbs are the action words, the strongest we have: *go*, *stop*, *admit*, *cut*, *discharge*. Every sentence needs a verb, which should be close to the subject noun in the sentence. Verbs can be expressed in active voice ("We found that...") or passive ("It was found that...").

Verbs also have tense—past, present, future, and variations thereof. There are two conventions in medical writing worth noting:

■ Within a scientific article, we use past tense to describe results:

> We found that one third of the rats survived, one third died, and the third rat got away.

■ In describing a published work, present tense is used:

> In their groundbreaking work, Smith and Jones report a 33% survival rate in the test population.

The infinitive is a verb form and in high school we were warned never, ever to split an infinitive. Today's custom allows a split infinitive if it will make the sentence clearer. For example:

■ Clumsy:

> Splitting an infinitive might greatly serve to clarify a sentence.

■ Better with a split infinitive:

> Splitting an infinitive might serve to greatly clarify a sentence.

Modifiers

Adjectives modify nouns and adverbs modify verbs, adjectives, and other adverbs. They are not strong words. Although judicious use can enrich your writing, beware the tendency to overuse modifiers. They creep into our writing easily, and beginning writers tend to overuse them. We use excessive modifiers in writing clinical notes ("well-developed, well-nourished, male factory worker in no acute distress") and sometimes we carry this over into our scientific writing. Here are two examples of sentences that string several modifiers together; the sentences contain all the necessary information, but lack strength. In the sentences, we lose the possible impact of any one of the modifiers, which might benefit from more discussion:

◼ Multiple adjectives:

> The patient was a tall, thin, anxious, elderly man.

◼ Multiple adverbs:

> The neurosurgeon operated skillfully, carefully, decisively, and seemingly effortlessly.

When you find yourself stringing several modifiers together, ask whether you need all of them. Do I really need all of the following adjectives?

> Peer reviewers found the article to be timely, interesting, scholarly, articulate, and comprehensive.

Metaphors and Similes

A metaphor is an implied comparison: "For the patient in the critical care unit, his wife's arrival at the bedside was always a ray of sunshine in his dull day." At the beginning of this chapter I wrote of ideas and structure as our blueprint, and paragraphs, sentences, and words as our tools. The words *blueprint* and *tools* used in this way represented metaphors. An explicit comparison is a simile: "A day without wine is like a day without sunshine."

We often use metaphors in medical writing, and some are embedded in our medical terminology: "coffee-ground vomitus," "cotton-wool exudates," "leonine facies," and "spider nevi." We say that a penetrating injury "invaded the abdominal cavity." Medical similes include poorly perfused feet that are "cold as ice" and the anemic patient whose skin appears "pale as a sheet."

Walt Kelly's Pogo said that, "Words are for people who can't read pictures." But words can be used to create pictures in our minds. Consider the following. Tobacco causes the deaths of 400,000 Americans each year. Big number. To be more specific, in the United States more than 1000 persons die each day of the effects of tobacco use. This has a little more punch. But try this word picture: The loss of life in the U.S. due to tobacco use is the equivalent of three jumbo jets crashing each day. For me, this image has vivid impact! Metaphors and similes enrich our writing, and the chief way we go wrong is mixing our images:

The dehydrated patient was bone-dry, like an old prune.

Onomatopoeia and Alliteration

Onomatopoeic words, also called echoic words, sound like the things they represent. In nature we have "cuckoo" and "whippoorwill." In medicine we find "hiccup," "murmur," "belch," "croup," and "cough." My favorite onomatopoeic word is *borborygmus*, which describes elephantine rumbling of the intestines. These words are generally short and strong, and sometimes colorful. When used correctly, they add vigor to your writing.

Alliteration, the repetition of the same letter or syllable in successive words, can be a different story. When writing I am often tempted to use alliteration, which appeals to my sense of play. But there is the reader to consider.

Alliteration almost always annoys an audience. The previous sentence, of course, is an example of alliteration. Some authors seem drawn to this form of expression, insisting that it provides emphasis. Experienced writers tend to purge alliteration from their manuscripts.

Eponyms

Diseases, anatomical structures, remedies, and other items named for famous physicians and scientists represent eponyms. The word itself comes from the Greek word *eponymas*, meaning "named after." Some of the many eponyms we all know include Bright's disease, tetralogy of Fallot, Graves' disease, Raynaud's syndrome, Hodgkin's disease, Hippocratic facies, and Paget's disease.

The current tendency is to replace these historic names with more scientific terms. Hence, von Recklinghausen's disease is now properly called neurofibromatosis, and Caffey's disease is infantile cortical hyperostosis. The astute medical writer should follow this lead in most cases, perhaps stating the accepted Greco-Latin phrase, followed by the historic eponym in parentheses—for example: relapsing febrile nodular nonsuppurative panniculitis (Weber-Christian disease).

Parenthetically, August Bier[7] once wrote: "When a disease is named after some author, it is very likely that we don't know much about it." The persistence of an eponym, such as Hodgkin's disease, might be a marker of a medical knowledge deficit. Might eponymic diseases be especially good topics for research studies and clinical articles?

Choosing the Words We Use

Words must be chosen with care. You should strive to use just the right word in the precise way. And you must try to avoid words that can annoy or confuse your reader.

Using Words Precisely

The following statement about a vaccine for traveler's diarrhea was published in November 2003. In my opinion, it has two errors. Can you find them?

> The new, one-dose vaccine is presently given in liquid form but could be developed in oral form.

Here they are: First, the word *presently* means soon, not now; the correct word in this instance should be *currently*. Second, is not a liquid also an oral form? I think that the author means to say that the new form will be a capsule or tablet.

Here are two other examples that found their way into print:

> He complained of numbness in his feet, which was gradually speeding proximally.

I believe that the author means that the numbness was spreading, not speeding.

> The incidence of uremic pericarditis occurs in 14–20% of patients undergoing dialysis.

This sentence is from one of America's leading medical journals. Incidence "is"; incidence does not "occur."

As you read medical journals in the months and years to come, look for small errors and imprecise word use. It will be amusing and will help make you a better writer.

Words that Might Annoy

Be sensitive to your audience. Do not call an anesthesiologist an anesthetist or refer to a family physician as a family practitioner. Never write about the orthopedic surgeon as an orthopod. Some of the words that arose as managed care jargon can irritate various clinicians, and writers should think twice before using them. Table 2.3 lists words that might grate on some readers.

TABLE 2.3. Annoying words (and abbreviations)

Words that may annoy	Why the word annoys some readers
Provider	Our readers are physicians, nurse practitioners, physician assistants, clinical psychologists and other clinicians. "Provider" is a lumping term that originated with third-party payers. Many are offended by this term, and the journal *America Family Physician* has specifically ceased its use.
PCP	This is supposed to refer to "primary care provider" or "primary care physician." The abbreviation can also stand for phencyclidine (phenylcyclohexyl piperidine) also called "angel dust," pulmonary capillary pressure, prochlorperazine, and *Pneumocystis carinii* pneumonia.
Covered lives	This phrase is another illegitimate child of the managed care payers. We treat patients, or perhaps clients if that is your discipline's preference. We do not care for "covered lives," a term that only dehumanizes those persons in our practices.
Mid-level provider	Nurse practitioners and physician assistants do not like this term, which is perceived as disrespectful.
Case	The sick person is a patient—or perhaps a man, woman, child, or person—but not a case. Cases are what lawyers argue in court.
Customer	Administrators like to talk about "customer service," as though we were selling used cars.

One consideration under the heading of possibly annoying words is what we call those who receive medical care. Throughout my career they have been patients. Recently, however, I have heard them called "clients." The recent emergence of "client" merits scrutiny. In part, at least, the word is an outgrowth of managed care, which helped bring us "provider" and "covered lives." It also may be the discipline-specific stylistic choice of some clinician-authors. Therefore, let us try to understand "client" vs. "patient" by going to the origins of the words.

"Patient" in English comes from Latin *pati* (to suffer), then Old French *pacient*, and later Middle English *pacyent*. The words have denoted a suffering person receiving medical care and that the person endured the illness calmly and with forbearance ("patience"). "Client," on the other hand, comes from the Anglo-French word *clyent*, meaning a person who is dependent on another. The word entered the English language to describe those who depended on lawyers, and later metamorphosed to include customers of other services. But not physicians. When I am next ill, I wish to be considered a patient and not a client.

Misused Words

Medical writers often misuse words. Sometimes it is hospital team conversation showing up in manuscripts. It may be an attempt to be "scientific." Perhaps the author is abusing the thesaurus. Examples of misused words include using *symptomatology* when we mean symptoms, using *impact* as a verb when the correct word would be *affect*, and dropping adverbs such as *hopefully* somewhere in an otherwise perfectly good sentence.

> Incorrect use: The patient hopefully will recover.
> Correct use: The clinicians and family all hope that the patient will recover.

All adverbs, most of which end in -ly, must modify a specific word that is not a noun. I hope that you will not allow adverbs such as *happily*, *sadly*, or *tragically* to wander about in your sentences like lost children.

TABLE 2.4. Words (and phrases) we misuse

Word or phrase	How we misuse the word
Data	This is a plural word. To write that "the data shows" is incorrect. The correct phrase is: "The data show…"
Presently	This word means soon, in a short time. Do not use "presently" when you mean to say "currently" or "now."
Mitigate	Mitigate means "to lessen in intensity or force." Thus it is wrong to say that an infusion of dextrose in water mitigated *against* the insulin-induced hypoglycemia. The addition of "against" is redundant and, in a sense, is a double negative.
Parameter	An arbitrary constant in a mathematical equation is a parameter. Other uses of this statistical term in scientific writing are generally incorrect.
Significant	When used in a scientific paper, this word had a statistical connotation.
Etiology	Remember that "-ology" at the end of any word means "the study of." Therefore, we should not write about *S. pneumoniae* as the "etiology" of pneumococcal pneumonia when we are really discussing the cause.
Very unique	This word means that there is only one (from Latin *unus*, meaning "one"). Thus, it is one of a kind or it is not, and no modifier is appropriate.
Equal halves	Halves cannot be unequal.

Table 2.4 lists some words that, I hope, you and I will not misuse in the future.

PUTTING IT TOGETHER

In this chapter, I have covered basic elements of article topic and organization, as well as issues in composing paragraphs, writing sentences, and selecting words. In the next chapter, I discuss putting it all together to create an article, with an eye to publication.

REFERENCES

1. Taylor RB. Learning to scramble. Fam Med 2001;33:629–630.
2. Taylor RB. How physicians read the medical literature. The Female Patient 2004;29(1):8–11.

3. Day RA. How to write and publish a scientific paper. 5th ed. Westport, CT: 1998:209.
4. Jordan EP, Shepard WC. Rx for medical writing. Philadelphia: WB Saunders; 1952:24.
5. Bernstein TM. The careful writer: a modern guide to English usage. New York: Atheneum; 1972:360.
6. Dirckx JH. The language of medicine. 2nd ed. New York: Praeger; 1983:85.
7. Bier A. Quoted in: Strauss MB. Familiar medical quotations. Boston: Little, Brown; 1968:116.

3

From Page One to the End

In Chapter 1, I reviewed your motivation to write, discussed how to find needed information, and considered the important questions that must be asked about any writing project. In Chapter 2, I discussed the blueprint for your project—the idea and structure—and the tools you will use, namely paragraphs, sentences, and words. Now let's look at putting it all together, from page one to the end, starting with your idea and how to handle to it.

CONCEPT AND STRUCTURE

You might begin with a nice focused topic such as "the new drug that cures the common cold: indications, administration, side effects and cost." Or perhaps you have just concluded the seminal study on whether or not eating rhubarb daily increases longevity; the medical world is awaiting the report and it is time to write up your results. Generally, however, your idea will be something like "the office approach to" acute sinusitis, back strain, or chronic pelvic pain.

With a general topic idea in mind, the next step is to limit the topic and find the best way to approach it. We discussed this briefly in Chapter 2. Because deciding on the concept and structure—how you will handle your topic—is so important, I will return to this process here, using the review article as a model.

Let us use sinusitis as an example of a very general topic. How might we limit the topic and organize an article? Logical questions are: Shall I write on pathophysiology, diagnosis, or treatment, or all three? Shall I write on acute or chronic sinusitis or both? Shall I cover adults or children or both? Is there any logic to covering women vs. men as patients? If covering treatment, should I include both medical and surgical therapy? How about herbal as well as traditional medical therapy? The following lists some of the article concepts possible with the general topic of sinusitis:

Pathophysiology:
    Microorganisms found in acute sinusitis
    Common precursors of acute sinusitis
    Complications of bacterial sinusitis
    Occupational issues in chronic sinusitis
    Chronic sinusitis in men and women: is there a difference?
    Causes of sinusitis in children and adolescents
Diagnosis:
    Recognizing bacterial sinusitis: common signs and symptoms
    Uncommon presentations of acute sinusitis
    Acute vs. chronic sinusitis: how to tell the difference
    When to image the patient with sinusitis
    Warning signs in the patient with acute sinusitis
Treatment:
    The best drugs to use in acute sinusitis
    Current surgical therapy of chronic sinusitis
    Herbal therapy of sinusitis
    Treating chronic sinusitis: an evidence-based approach
    Managing chronic sinusitis: treatments that do not work
    When to refer the patient with sinusitis

Any symptom, sign, or diagnosis in medicine can yield many ideas for an article. Here is a useful exercise. Pick a general area—such as skin rash, abdominal pain, or pneumonia—that interests you, and then think of at least 15 ways to write a review article about this topic.

If there is one aspect of an article you want to get just right, it is how you deal with your topic. A copyeditor can correct spelling, fix grammatical errors, and untangle tortuous syntax. But a copyeditor cannot fix structure. Think of a house: copyediting represents redecorating. Structural change, moving walls and raising roofs, is much more ambitious. Because finding the best concept and structure for the article is so important, I will return to the topic again in Chapter 6. Here I will present some actual published articles and examine how the authors dealt with their topics.

After selecting a focused topic and deciding on a structural concept, the experienced writer embarks on a "gestational period" during which the idea is pondered from various approaches, thinking about cases, lists, headings, examples from personal experience, and what really should be shared with the reader. During the gestational time, you will collect and organize data that will be needed for your paper.

COLLECTING AND ORGANIZING DATA

The "data phase" is important because it provides the basic facts you will present in your article. You will need these facts—for example, in a headache article I may tell that migraine headaches affect 18 percent of women and 6 percent of men during their lifetimes—when you begin to actually write. Not having necessary data at hand will break your creative train of thought, possibly with terrible consequences.

What you need before you start writing varies a little with the type of article or book chapter you are writing. I will cover the differences later as we discuss writing case reports, editorials, reports of original research, and so forth. However, for all articles you will need your basic research tools, notes, outline, and references.

Basic Research Tools

Every writer's research tools were discussed in Chapter 1. To review, these included a computer with a word processing program, medical dictionary, classic specialty-specific reference book, and access to Web sites described on pages 14–22. Here I want to discuss one more information collection tool: network research. Let's assume that I want to learn how many parking spaces are in the parking lots at Portland International Airport. I would start by calling someone in the airport administrative offices, who will refer me to someone who knows about parking, and then this person will know some more specifics about the various lots. I would wager that I could get the exact answer by the seventh telephone call. This is network research.

If I wanted to find out whether someone is working on the brilliant research question I just dreamed up, I would embark on some network research. I would search PubMed, MDConsult, or Google to find out who has written on the topic recently. Then I would turn to the telephone or e-mail. My favorite question is: "Who could I contact that might know more about this topic?"

Notes

How you save and organize your notes is very personal, and your method is very likely to change over time. After all, few today use 3- by 5-inch index cards any more.

In preparing this book, I have used a combination of paper and computer. For my research, I have photocopied article and book pages. I have also printed computer screens. For each of these paper documents, I have been careful to include the full identification of the source. For photocopied articles and book pages, this is easily accomplished by creating a small piece of paper telling the source and then putting this on the photocopy screen so that it is copied onto each page. Printouts of Web pages come with the Web site identified. I believe that including the full source on every note page is important to help avoid confusion about the source of ideas and phrases. It is much too easy to become an accidental plagiarist if you make notes without careful attribution. (More about plagiarism in Chapter 5.)

Notes include personal "bright ideas." These can come at any time, and getting them in your notes can be like catching a sunbeam. Your "bright idea" notes can be recorded on paper, or, as I have done in working on these chapters, added to a Microsoft (MS) Word document labeled "Booknotes.doc." I arrange these "bright idea" notes by chapter. Then as I begin work on a new chapter, I "cut and paste" the notes into the first draft, thereby avoiding retyping.

I suggest that you be expansive in assembling notes. What seems not pertinent today may be an idea that proves useful later. After you complete your project, what was not used can be discarded or saved for another project. Also, note that in the end, more than half your notes will probably not be used, at least in the current project.

Outline

As you have already discovered, I am an outline advocate. I like to determine the topic and concept first, and then think about the general structure of the article. For example, assume that you are writing an article on the general topic of edema. The concept might be "five uncommon causes of edema." Then the outline's major headings could be:

> Abstract
> Background
> Selected Causes
> Clinical Significance
> References

From here you might expand the outline to the next level of headings:

> Abstract
> Background
>   Epidemiology
>   Definitions
>   Why the issue is important
> Selected Causes
>   Hypothyroidism
>   Sodium overload
>   Hypoalbuminemia
>   Cyclic edema in women
>   Medication use
> Clinical Significance
>   When to consider an uncommon cause
>   What is important in daily practice?
> References

After taking notes and thinking about the topic, you might further expand the outline to include topics to be covered under each subheading:

Abstract
> This will be a summary of the main sections: background, the five selected causes of edema, and the clinical significance of these causes.

Background
> Epidemiology
>> How often do we see patients with unexplained edema?
>> What clinicians are likely to see these patients?
>
> Definitions: "localized" vs. "generalized" edema
> Why the issue is important
>> Value of early therapy
>> Dangers of missed diagnoses

Selected Causes (give presentation and diagnostic features of each)
> Hypothyroidism
> Sodium overload
> Hypoalbuminemia
>> Malnutrition
>> Cirrhosis of the liver
>> Nephrotic syndrome
>> Protein-losing enteropathy
>
> Cyclic edema in women
> Medication use
>> Nonsteroidal antiinflammatory drugs, estrogens, corticosteroids, antihypertensives, and others

Clinical Significance
> When to consider an uncommon cause
> What is important in daily practice?

References

You can see how the expanded outline grows. It will be very useful when you write the first draft because you will already have made many of the critical decisions. With that said, I want to say a word about flexibility. It is important that the outline does not become a straitjacket. Be willing to modify and enhance your plan. New ideas will emerge as you write, and sometimes will be good enough to prompt a change in the outline. I always hope that the change is minor (redecorating) rather than major (moving a weight-bearing wall). Embarking on a structural change when halfway through the first draft is, at best, a frustrating activity.

References

Managing references during article preparation is an art. There are many ways to manage references, and the method you choose will vary with the number of references in your article or book chapter. If your article has relatively few references, fewer than 20, I think it is acceptable to use the method I have used in each of these chapters. First, remember that each page of notes should contain the full reference source. Then as I type a sentence that calls for a reference citation, I type the full source in parentheses at the end of the sentence, and put it in bold font so I can find it easily later. It looks like this:

> ...so I can find it easily later. **(Taylor RB. The clinician's guide to medical writing. New York: Springer-Verlag; 2005: 67.)**

Then I continue to write and revise successive drafts. At the end, when I consider the article or chapter almost done— and beyond any major changes—I substitute sequential numbers for the references, and I move the citations to the reference list using the MS Word "cut and paste" feature. In the end, the manuscript sentence will be:

> ...It looks like this.[1]

The method may seem a little primitive, but it works well for me, perhaps because my writing rarely has a large number of reference citations.

Another way to manage references is the use of EndNote software. This sophisticated program allows users to search online bibliographic databases and to keep track of their references. Once you have mastered its use, you can create and edit bibliographies readily. The disadvantages are cost (currently more than $150 for the full product) and the steep learning curve facing the new user. The program is not "intuitive" and the online instructions are ponderous. You can learn more about EndNote software by starting with www.google.com, searching "Endnote," and then following the trail.

EndNote software is great for experienced and prolific medical authors, especially if compiling long lists of citations. However, in my opinion, beginning medical authors should use my more primitive "cut and paste" method, and spend their energy learning how to be better writers.

How Much Preparation is Enough?

It is possible to overprepare to write. Some authors seem to become mired in the data collection phase and never emerge. Do not overprepare. When you have your research tools, notes, outline, and references all together, the time has come to begin the first draft.

BEGINNING: THE FIRST DRAFT

Getting Started

Setting the Stage

Do not begin to write the first draft until you have set the stage. Yes, you already have your research tools, notes, and so forth, but there is one more thing you will need for an outstanding first draft: uninterrupted time. Collecting data, constructing an outline, and later revising are all important grunt work that can be accomplished in discontinuous periods of time. This is not true of writing the first draft, which is the truly creative part of the work. For this effort, you will need several hours of uninterrupted time. (See Chapter 1 for some hints on how to find this elusive time.) For the average length article and with adequate preparation, you should plan on 2 to 3 hours to create the first draft. When writing a first draft, I have joked to my colleagues that, if interrupted, when I open the door I expect to see flames in the hallway.

Not being interrupted also means not stopping to look things up. The first draft is about getting your thoughts down on paper in a logically organized way. It is not about spelling, minor grammatical errors, or best word choice. Do not stop writing to look things up online; this can come later in the revision phase.

Where and How to Begin

When faced with an empty computer screen, what do you do next? For both beginning and experienced authors, getting the first few words in type can be the most difficult step in writing. Jordan and Shepard[2] state, "The first few words are like a plunge into an ice cold pool. It isn't so bad after the start has been made."

Here are some good ways to get started:

■ Start at the very beginning and keep going until you are finished. Some very experienced authors can do this, and can accurately estimate the length of the finished article. I admire these gifted individuals, and hope someday to achieve this exalted state.

■ Expand the outline with chunks of words, jumping about as the spirit moves you. In the edema article outlined above, I might write a paragraph about a patient I saw with edema, and then another paragraph covering how sodium overload occurs and how it may be recognized. In the end, I will fit these disparate bits and pieces together like a jigsaw puzzle, using the planned structure, to create a draft of the article.

■ Create the tables and figures. This is one of my favorite methods. Many articles and book chapters are built around one or more tables. Creating these tables—making decisions on column headings and what to include—can bring clarity to the entire piece you are writing. In writing this book, I first assembled my expanded outline and notes. My next step was to create the tables for each chapter, all the way to the end of the book.

■ Write the abstract. In general, I advise writing the abstract last. After all, it is a synopsis of the article, and you won't really know the full content of the article until it is done. But when at a loss for a beginning, writing a tentative synopsis can focus your thinking and get some words on paper.

■ Answer the WIRMS question: What I Really Mean to Say is... If having trouble getting started, answer the WIRMS question in one to three sentences, and see if this starts the flow of words.

Delaying Tactics

At this point, I want to talk about delaying tactics. When it is time to sit down and write, almost any other activity seems to be more interesting or urgent. My favorite delaying tactics are getting coffee, surfing the Web in search of one more nugget of information, or rearranging items on my desk. For others, they are making a telephone call or answering e-mail messages—anything but engaging the brain and writing.

For some authors, actions such as sharpening a handful of pencils are actually rituals that signal them that it is time to write. For others the activities are impediments to writing, and should be recognized for the undesirable behavior they represent.

Words One, Two, and Beyond

The actual opening sentence of a paper is important, first to get words on the screen, and second to set the tone for the article. The first sentence often states the problem in general terms. For example, "Unexplained edema can be a diagnostic challenge." Or, "Osteoporosis is a common problem of women over age 60."

An alternative opening for an article or book chapter is to present a clinical vignette: "The patient was a 48-year-old woman, in otherwise good health, with swelling of the feet and hands for more than 6 months." Such a first sentence piques the interest of most clinicians.

Whatever the first sentence, the beginning of an article should set the stage and get the article moving. Not all articles begin with the general, unassailable statement. Table 3.1 lists examples of other ways to start an article or a chapter.

Getting Stuck

At some time while writing the early drafts, you are likely to get stuck. The words just won't come. You look out the window, go out for the mail, or play with the dog. You engage in all the delaying tactics listed above. You wonder if you are

TABLE 3.1. Some ways to begin an article or chapter

The beginning	Example
Purpose of the article	This paper presents an evidence-based approach to the management of the common cold.
Scope of the article	This paper discusses five causes of generalized edema.
Viewpoint of the paper	Calling clinicians "providers" insults our professionalism.
Quotation from a respected source	In a recent report in *Lancet*, Smith et al report that . . .
Framing a question	What is the best way to reduce teen pregnancy?
Positing an argument to be refuted	Flu shots are not given in the first trimester of pregnancy. Is this logical?
Focus on action	Now is the time for physicians to speak out on the proposed changes in Medicare.
Compare and contrast	Some physicians prescribe antibiotics empirically for adult patients with acute bronchitis manifested as fever and severe cough. Others do not.
Beginning with a question	The next patient you see may have pertussis. Will you recognize the symptoms and signs?
The startling statistic	Up to one third of Americans with hypertension are undiagnosed, and only about half of those known to have hypertension are adequately controlled.

having a TIA (transient ischemic attack, a small stroke). Face it. You have writer's block, a temporary affliction that affects every author eventually. Perhaps the causes relate to the fear of others criticizing your work; maybe you suffer from excessive self-criticism. Or, for the time being, you are out of words.

Here are some methods to help get unstuck:

■ Brainstorm the main idea. Forget your careful outline for a while. Write down lots of new ideas about your topic. Expand a few of them. Can you think of cases to use as examples?
■ Revisit the outline. Go to each main heading and write down what you mean to present in each section. Expand the outline to include some phrases you will use in the actual writing.

- Review your notes. Add new ideas, maybe short paragraphs, as they occur to you. Add examples and quotes.
- Leapfrog. Stop trying to write sequentially. Jump around in your draft to the next section that interests you. Then fill in the gaps later.
- Change your writing method for a while. Leave your computer and use pen and paper.
- Reread what you have done so far. As you look over what you have written, maybe new ideas will come to you.
- Change your writing time. We are almost all morning or evening people, and probably write during our best time. If stuck, try writing during your "off time." That is, if you are a morning person, try writing in the evening for a while.
- Prepare a lecture. Imagine that you must present your paper to colleagues tomorrow morning. How would you organize and present the information?
- Talk to a colleague. Discussing your project with an insightful coworker can help bring out the ideas hiding just below the surface.
- Rewrite. If desperate, try rewriting a key section of what you have already written.
- Rest your mind. If all else fails, try delaying tactics that actually rest your mind. Take a walk, listen to classical music, watch football on television, or meditate.

Eventually you will get unstuck, and you will finish the first draft. Next comes the less creative, more tedious, but very essential task—revision.

THE MIDDLE: REVISING YOUR WORK

Revision, editing your own work, may seem like extracting your own impacted molar. It must be done, but it can be painful. The analogy of this editing and tooth extraction is appropriate because of the origins of the word *edit*. This word comes from Latin words *dare*, meaning "to give" and *e*, meaning "out." In Latin these root words gave *editus*, meaning "to put out."[3] Thus, the editing function is chiefly one of "putting out," and this is especially true of revising (editing your own work).

There is, however, one major difference between revising (removing your own molar) and editing (having the procedure performed by someone who probably has more skill than you). King,[4] an experienced editor, describes this difference very well: "If, when engaged in editing, you feel that major changes are in order, you cannot be sure that any alterations you propose will express what the author wanted to say. You may be distorting his meaning. In revision, however, you are in control at all times. You have complete freedom to make all the changes you want."

There are probably as many ways of revising as there are writers. With that said, I wish to consider some principles. The first principle is the number of revisions. The astute reader has noted that the previous section of the chapter was titled "Beginning: The First Draft." An article should undergo at least three preliminary drafts before the final version. In performing the three pre-final drafts, you may choose to follow this pattern:

- *First revision*: In the first look at your creative first draft, look at the "wholeness" of the paper. At this stage, try not to be too focused on minor errors of spelling and grammar. Instead, verify that your structure is sound and that what you say is really appropriate for your intended audience and the target journal (or the edited book, if writing a book chapter). It is okay to fix the level of a heading or two, but the emphasis must be on reviewing the organization, logic, and validity of what you have written. Does it all hang together? Have I said what I wanted to say?

- *Second revision*: The second time through the manuscript is when you verify. Look for errors in spelling, grammar, and syntax. Check carefully for factual errors. Be sure to run your Microsoft (MS) Word spelling and grammar checker, but do not rely on it; the spell checker may accept "of" when you meant to type "for." If a sentence or paragraph is in the wrong location, now is the time to move it. If a heading is needed, insert it now. If you find superfluous phrases or wordy constructions, eliminate them.

- *Third revision*: By now you have checked for any major problems, and repaired minor errors. Before undertaking the next revision, it is a good idea to put the paper away for a week or two. This cooling-off period will "disconnect" you from the writing, and when you read the paper again, you will often wonder, How could I have ever written this sentence?

In the third revision, you vigorously polish your work to make it shine. The emphasis here is on clarity and style. You will simplify words, seek the best way to express your thoughts, and eliminate unnecessary verbiage. You will also be looking for danger signs: inappropriate stance, favored but inappropriate phrases, and cuteness.

Style and Clarity

Style, in writing, describes the way ideas are expressed. It has to do with word selection, how the words are arranged into sentences, and how the sentences are linked together to create paragraphs. Whether or not quotes and borrowed material are used are elements of style. Style includes the use or absence of humor, playfulness, and even one's self in the writing. I consider style the fingerprints of the author. As an editor of multiauthor reference books, I have received some manuscripts created by two or three authors. If one author wrote the first half and author number two the second, I can tell when authorship changes within the chapter, even if the manuscript has the same font throughout. I can tell the shift in authorship because the style abruptly changes.

Norton[5] said, "Remember that a straightforward and unadorned writing style has its own elegance." We should all strive for the style Norton describes, clear exposition of ideas, written in the smallest words and cleanest sentences possible. If such writing seems a little bland, it can be flavored with some variety in word choice, alternatively constructed sentences, and a few carefully selected quotations.

Clarity means clearness, and in writing it refers to simple, direct expression of ideas. In medical writing, clarity is often the victim of completeness. How often do we read convoluted sentences with abundant phrases strung together just so that everything is included before getting to the terminal period?

Such convolution is most often seen in the results section of the abstract, but can occur anywhere in a medical article. Just to illustrate what I mean, here is a sentence that is complete, but is less than crystal-clear:

> As they begin to study medicine, and especially the pathogenesis and early manifestations of disease, medical students are likely to be taught by lecturers that use the same notes from year to year, prompting complaints that the teaching is not responsive to advances in clinical practice, but on the other hand, delighting the students who can purchase typed notes from members of previous classes, feeling secure in the knowledge that the lecture content has not changed, and allowing them to skip classes, while studying for examinations from notes that might otherwise be considered outdated if only the professor updated the content a little each year.

Whew! It is okay to breathe now. My trusty MS Word spelling and grammar checker did not highlight this sentence as being too long.

Weighty Words and Sentences

Good style calls for careful word selection. During revision, you should seek all the heavyweight words in your article and, whenever possible, replace them with those that are shorter and perhaps less "Latinized." Doing so will make your article easier to read (style) and understand (clarity). To do this, you must substitute *use* for *utilize* and *first* for *initial*. Table 3.2 lists some weighty words and good choices to replace them.

Alternative Ways to Express Your Thoughts

Experienced writers have a bank of alternative words and constructions to express their thoughts. The beginning writer does also, but in a different location. For the experienced author, the reservoir is in his or her head, deposited there by years of experience. For the neophyte, the reservoir is the thesaurus, whether a book or as part of the MS Word program. I will first discuss alternative forms of expression, and then the use and misuse of the thesaurus.

TABLE 3.2. Selected heavyweight words and suggested replacements

Heavyweight word	Good choice as a replacement
Initiate	Start, begin
Terminate	Stop, end
Sufficient	Enough
Perform	Do
Ultimate	Last
Transpire	Happen
Individual	Person
Institution	Hospital
Predominate	Chief
Etiology	Cause
Numerous	Many
Diminutive	Small

In the last paragraph, I wrote of the "beginning writer" in the second sentence, and then referred to this person again in the fourth sentence. To avoid using the term *beginning writer* again, I used the word *neophyte*. In sentences one and two I used the word *writer*, and in sentence three *author* was substituted. These are alternative words.

In the paragraph just above are two alternative constructions. Can you find them?

In the first sentence "wrote of" in the first part of the sentence became "referred to" in the second part. In the third sentence the active tense "I used the word" alternates with the passive "was substituted."

I must speak sternly about thesaurus use and abuse. Properly used, the thesaurus is an excellent source of synonyms and can give a list alternative words when you find yourself using favorite words repeatedly. For example, searching my MS Word thesaurus for "word" yielded the following:

Utterance
Sound
Statement
Expression
Speech
Remark
Declaration

Changing the search to the plural form "words" gave a very different list:

Language
Vocabulary
Terms
Expressions
Terminology
Lexis (Yes, lexis: It is really there.)

After reviewing the lists for alternatives to *word*, I might select *statement* or *expression* from the first list, and *term* from the second list. I probably would not use *utterance*, which seems to connote verbal, not written, expression. And the word *lexis* sounds like the name of an expensive car.

On the other hand, it is possible to misuse the thesaurus. By consulting the thesaurus for synonyms for only three words, this simple sentence,

The patient had a dull pain in the low back.

might become

The patient had an uninteresting hurting in the low rear.

The opportunities for malapropisms are endless. I call the act of consulting a thesaurus to find a complex word to replace a short one "thesaurus abuse." This is a new term, and you read it here first. I hope that no reader of this book engages in this nefarious practice, and that you resolve today to use the thesaurus only to seek the best word and appropriate alternative ways to express your ideas.

Removing Stuff

If you are like me, your first draft is chock full of stuff, bursting like an overfilled Christmas stocking. The stuff—items typed because you wisely did not stop your creative act to ponder best words and sentence structure—needs to be débrided during revision. Remember from above that much editing is "taking out" stuff.

A favorite writing principle is called *Occam's razor*. William of Occam was an English philosopher and theologian who lived in the 14th century, and held the enviable title of Doctor Invincibilis and Venerabilis. The Occam's razor principle arose with his statement, "Entities [he was referring to assumptions used to explain things] should not be multiplied beyond what is needed."[6] According to this dictum, you should "shave off" anything superfluous to the core message. Say only what is needed and no more. That applies to unnecessary words, paragraphs, and even sections of an article.

Removing Words
Good candidates for removal are instances of "doubling." This occurs when you use two words with virtually identical meaning to express the same thought. Some examples that show that saying it twice is not better than saying it once are:

> This is my *last* and *final* offer.

> She had a *life-threatening* and *potentially fatal* disease.

> The physician was *concerned* and *worried* about the patient's progress.

Other words begging to be removed are strings of adjectives or adverbs and long ponderous phrases. Consider how the following awkward sentence can be simplified:

> The patient was admitted to the hospital for the express purpose of ruling out the admittedly somewhat remote possibility that he might have pancreatic cancer.

Removing Paragraphs and Sections of the Article
Sometimes you must remove entire paragraphs and sections, or perhaps move one to another location. The removal process is usually prompted by one of two events: First, you realize that the paragraph is inappropriate, irrelevant to the core of the paper, or perhaps illogical, silly, or contradictory to something appearing elsewhere in the paper. In such instances, removal is needed. Second, the journal editor mandates that your 20-page paper be shortened to 10 pages.

In such instances, you are unlikely to find that half your words can be eliminated by fine-tuning sentences one by one. In such a case, major surgery is required, and you will probably need to eliminate one or more parts of the article.

Danger Signs

In revising your drafts, be alert for danger signs: red-flag phrases, the phrase that warms your heart, and cuteness.

Red-Flag Phrases

We all recognize a red flag as a sign of danger. Possible trouble lies ahead. A red-flag phrase is what I call a cluster of words that should warn you, during revision, that you might be getting into trouble. You may be about to write something that will undermine the credibility of your article or invite criticism by experts in the field. You may even be exposing that you could have dug more deeply during your research phase, or spent more time analyzing data. Table 3.3 lists my favorite red-flag phrases.

TABLE 3.3. Red-flag phrases

Red-flag phrase	Tongue-in-cheek translation
There are no prior published studies on the topic of . . .	Actually, I didn't spend much time searching the literature.
Authorities agree that . . .	We discussed this over coffee.
It is well known that . . .	I think I am right about this.
One can reasonably assume that . . .	I really hope that what I am about to say is true.
It is interesting to note that . . .	At least I think it is interesting.
The data clearly show that . . .	My intuition makes me believe that what I am about to write is correct.
It is evident that . . .	Ditto above, and my statistics are shaky.
In other words . . .	I am about to repeat myself.
Based on the results presented, practicing clinicians should . . .	My way or the highway! Trial attorneys love this language.
Further studies are required to further investigate . . .	I need another research grant.

The Phrase that Warms Your Heart

Sometimes you will find a wonderful phrase (or sentence) and you just must get it in. You may believe that you have found the odd fact during your research, and even though it is superfluous to your research, you really want to get it in your report. This is generally a signal that you should take it out.

Someday you may even be tempted to include a phrase that, to those in the know, is a subtle personal attack on a rival. Such thoughts should never even occur on your monitor screen.

Other candidates are the instances of alliteration as discussed in Chapter 2, which sound so good in your head, and read so poorly. Also consider eliminating the tendency to "name something." As I type this, I am considering taking out the term red-flag phrases above, but I decided that the title of the table has value. I hope this turns out to be a good decision.

Cuteness

I began Chapter 1 by asserting that being a good clinician does not make one a capable writer. It also does not make one humorous. Most of us are not actually as funny as we think, and writing humor is especially difficult because you don't have available the inflections and timing that help make stories funny. Thus when you and I attempt humor we often become "cute." Cuteness in a medical article is terrible.

"You can observe a lot by just watching." One way beginning writers introduce cuteness is the beginning quotation—the Yogi Berra expression or the passage from the Peanuts comic strip found at the beginning of an article or chapter. Sometimes using such quotations enhances your writing, especially when a Yogi Berra aphorism or a passage from Shakespeare is woven into the subsequent prose.

Of course, some levity can make reading more enjoyable. A few pages ago, in discussing thesaurus use, I quipped about the word *lexis* sounding like an expensive car (even though the spelling of the car name is Lexus), and in Table 3.3 I created fanciful translations of the worrisome phrases. Did these attempts at wit work for you or not? If not, please consider them to be planned examples of what not to do.

The Colleague as a Critical Reader

When you have finished at least three revisions and are almost ready to prepare the final draft, it is time to pass the manuscript to a colleague for critical review. The process is sometimes called "informal refereeing." If your critical reader does the job you expect, you will learn at least some of the weaknesses in your paper and be able to correct them before submission to your target journal. Believe an experienced writer when I say that it is much better to find the manuscript's flaws before it leaves my office than to have the errors discovered by the journal's peer reviewers and thereby trigger rejection by the very journal that I most wanted to publish the paper.

What are the characteristics of the critical reader? This colleague must understand the science involved and know the principles of good writing. More important, the critical reader must not be intimidated or overly impressed with your writing skills. Reading the article and reporting "This is excellent" is no help at all. You need someone who is tough, honest, and not afraid to use the red pen liberally. Among medical writers, this has been called "benign brutality." Of course, there is the understanding that, when your critical reader is writing an article, you will provide a reciprocal reading.

Must the critical reader be a clinician in your same specialty? No. In the past an excellent critical reader was a nurse practitioner faculty member who was also a prolific author. I have served as critical reader for a gynecologic oncologist who was an international medical graduate and whose English language skills lacked some of the subtleties needed for precise written prose. A nonmedical person may also review the article, looking for clear English and logical development of the message. For decades, my best critical reader has been my wife, who is a successful author in her own right.

Instructions for the critical reader are important. You are not asking for redaction—the process of word-by-word, sentence-by-sentence editing. And you do not merely wish for general comments. Here are some specific questions for the critical reader:

- Can you state in one sentence what the article is trying to say?

■ Is what I am saying medically (or scientifically) sound?
■ Are there any errors of fact?
■ Should the structure be changed in some way?
■ Is my prose clear?
■ How can the article be improved?

GETTING FINISHED: THE FINAL DRAFT

There is no perfect paper. There will never be one. No paper can be perfect because writers, readers, and reviewers have different ideas about content, structure, and style. All writing can be criticized as too broad or narrow, too elementary or complex, too long or too short. At only 266 words, the Gettysburg address was criticized in its day.

Certainly, each of us should aim for excellence, and should revise as needed—within limits. It is interesting to note that Ernest Hemingway revised the last page of *A Farewell to Arms* 39 times.[7] Rachel Carson, author of *The Sea Around Us* (1951) and *Silent Spring* (1962), said that writing is "largely a matter of application and hard work, of writing and rewriting endlessly until you are satisfied that you have said what you want to say as clearly and simply as possible." She states that for her that means "many, many revisions."[8]

On the other hand, you must eventually finish, as did Hemingway and Carson. In the quest for the final draft, do not let perfect become the enemy of the good. There will come a time when you must say, "This is as good as I can make it."

Once, when I was quite young, I spent a summer selling cars. I learned soon that I earned no commission unless I could close the deal. To earn a paycheck, I learned to be a "closer." That is, I learned to get the job done, signed, delivered. In medical writing, this means declaring the manuscript done and sending it off.

Completing a manuscript and letting it go is not easy for some. Some of the excuses for late manuscripts that I have received are presented in Table 3.4.

There are some ways to help you finish the job. One is to establish a deadline: I will definitely finish the article and get it mailed before the end of the month. Then stick to this deadline,

TABLE 3.4. Excuses that have been offered for late or missing manuscripts

Illness or injury: A wide variety was reported in authors and their families. These included nervous breakdown, depression, cancer, auto accidents, and more.

Divorce: "My wife has left me and I don't know what I am going to do. But I am sure I will not get the book chapter done."

Technical problems: "I was almost done and then my computer crashed, and I had not backed up the file."

An act of God: "We had a fire in our house and the manuscript burned."

Blame the other guy: "My coauthor hasn't completed his half of the manuscript yet."

Job change, especially when it was involuntary: "Dr. Smith doesn't work here anymore, and I don't know where she might be."

I have to pay the light bill: "Sorry, but I am way behind on writing grants, which I need to support my salary."

A report from the administrative assistant: "Dr. Jones is away at a conference again. I don't know anything about a manuscript."

Academy Award excuse: "The manuscript was washed away by a flood."

My favorite: "You weren't really serious about a deadline, were you?"

even if you must work evenings and weekends. Another method to reach closure is to establish a reward goal: When I finish and mail the manuscript, I will take a long weekend and go to the beach.

If you are very lucky, you have the inherent ability to call a halt at just the right time, and declare, "It is done." You will mail the manuscript and await a reply, hoping for the best. In reality, most beginning medical writers will experience a number of rejections. You should consider these negative responses valuable, and free, lessons in learning your writing craft.

The potential for rejection in the peer-review process is just one of the features that are special about medical writing. In the next chapter, I will discuss some technical issues that are important when clinicians write for the medical literature.

REFERENCES

1. Taylor RB. The clinician's guide to medical writing. New York: Springer-Verlag; 2005:67.
2. Jordan EP, Shepard WC. Rx for medical writing. Philadelphia: WB Saunders; 1952:7.

3. Partridge E. Origins: a short etymological dictionary of modern English. New York: Macmillan; 1966:177.
4. King LS. Why not say it clearly? Boston: Little, Brown; 1978:97.
5. Norton SA. Read this but skip that. J Am Acad Dermatol 2001;44:714–715.
6. Benet WR. Reader's encyclopedia. 3rd ed. New York: Harper & Row; 1987:706.
7. Plimpton G. Writers at work. New York: Viking Press; 1963:124.
8. Brooks P. The house of life: Rachel Carson at work. Boston: Houghton, Mifflin; 1972:1–3.

4

Technical Issues in Medical Writing

In contrast to the past three chapters, which have covered the concept and prose aspects of medical writing, this chapter addresses some technical issues you will face. Do not, however, think that constructing tables and figures is any less creative than composing words and sentences; in fact, developing these supplements to the text may be the most innovative part of writing your article. Other technical issues—such as copyright, permissions, and reference citations—may become important as you seek publication of your work.

TABLES

Tables are lists of words and numbers; they do not contain artwork. If what you are presenting includes a drawing, photograph, or diagonal lines that connect data (such as an algorithm), it is a figure (see Figures, below).

Tables, a useful device in preparing an article or a book chapter, offer the following advantages:

- *Presenting data*: A table is usually the best way to arrange numerical data groups or lists.
- *Combining words and numbers*: Tables allow the clean presentation of combinations of words and numerical data.
- *Avoiding unintelligible complex sentences*: A table is better than a long list of items in a 75-word sentence.
- *Breaking up the flow of text*: Tables allow some variety in the appearance of your article by introducing some white space on the page.

There are two types of table—the so-called text table and the more formal table. The list in the last paragraph (about the advantages of tables) is a text table. In fits nicely into the flow of prose and it introduces some variety into how information is presented. Text tables should be logical lists and must be relatively short. Because they are integrated into the flow of the paragraph, no citation (such as see Table 1.1) is needed.

Formal tables are separated from the written paragraphs, and are cited in the text. Table 4.1, which lists the characteristics of a good table, is an example of a formal table.

About Tables

In many articles, the table is the key feature of what you want to present. For example, if you wished to present the presenting symptoms, signs, diagnostic criteria, and treatment of common childhood infections, a table would be an economical way to do so. In this instance, I would construct the table before beginning to write the prose.

Every table must have a title that describes its content, and the table with its title should stand alone. I tell students that

TABLE 4.1. Characteristics of a good table

Characteristic	What I mean to say is...
Not too long or wide	The ideal table fits on a single journal or book page. Tables that run over to a second or even third page are difficult for the printer to fit into the publication and for the reader to follow.
Clearly written title	The title makes sense without referring back to the text.
Not too much text	If you are inserting long paragraphs into a table, maybe the information should be in the text and you don't need a table at all.
Not too many columns	Probably the ideal table has three to five columns. More than five columns may be needed, but sometimes at the expense of easy reading.
All abbreviations explained in the table footnote	Even if the abbreviations are explained in the text, be kind to your reader and present what they represent again in the table footnote.
Not too many abbreviations	Excessive use of abbreviations can compromise readability; this is especially true in a table.
Not too many footnotes	As a reader, I don't like jumping from table to footnotes and back.

a reader speaking on your topic, such as childhood infections or headache, should be able to make your table directly into a PowerPoint slide and have it make sense. Thus, all abbreviations used must be explained in the table, either in the table footnote or in the table itself.

Tables must not duplicate what is written in the text. In Table 4.1 I list the characteristics of a good table. I should not repeat the points made in the table, although I might expand on one or two in the text.

When it comes to borrowing items from existing publications, tables are like artwork. No matter how short the table, if you wish to borrow a published table for use in your article, you need written permission. You also need permission if you "adapt" a published table or combine data from existing tables into what seems to be your own table. For these reasons, I advise authors to create their own tables whenever possible. In this book, there are no borrowed tables.

In editing book chapters, I find that tables are especially prone to errors in print. One reason that tables are error-magnets lies in the difficulty of constructing a table and communicating this through the editing and printing process. I have found many errors introduced during "mark-up" at the hands of copyeditors and typesetters who, understandably, do not know the medical meaning of what is in the table. Then things continue during proofreading. When reading proofs, authors seem to focus on the prose and forget to read the tables carefully, allowing errors to slip through. The more complex and data-laden the table, the more the author seems reluctant to proofread it carefully.

What Journal Editors Want

Tables must have titles (legends) and each column must have a short heading. If the table is borrowed, the source should be identified in the table footnote according to the style of the journal. Tables must be numbered in the order in which they are cited in the text. All tables should be double-spaced, even though this creates tables that extend to several manuscript pages.

Do not use too many tables in your article, because this may cause difficulty in page layout. I recently reviewed an article with nine manuscript pages and 10 tables. I advised the author to find a way to do without at least half the tables.

If you must use footnotes, consult the journal's instructions for authors to find the journal's preferred footnote symbols and sequence.

Submitting Tables

When submitting a paper manuscript, each table should be submitted on separate pages. This is done because, in preparing your manuscript for publication, tables (and figures) are often handled differently from prose. If a table is continued on subsequent manuscript pages, repeat the title on each page and cite the page number for the table (e.g., Table 4.1. Characteristics of a good table, page 2, page 3, etc.).

The *Journal of the American Medical Association* (JAMA) requests that authors copy all tables onto the disk to be submitted electronically or at the end of the text document for electronic submissions.[1]

Camera-Ready Copy

One way to minimize errors in your tables is to submit camera-ready tables. Camera-ready tables are created on your computer and then are reproduced photographically. This helps you as the author, because you avoid the painstaking task of proofreading the tables. Copyeditors cannot change your camera-ready table, which sometimes may be disadvantageous when an error is found. Publishers like camera-ready copy of all types, since it reduces production costs. If you are considering submitting camera-ready tables, consult the journal's instructions to authors or call the editor.

FIGURES

Charles Dickens, Jane Austen, and James Joyce did not need to worry about figures. Neither do Tom Clancy or Maya Angelou. In fact, few authors in history have included illustrations in their work. One exception was Lewis Carroll, who illustrated *Through the Looking Glass* with figures that he drew himself. The medical historians among us may be interested to know that Carroll was a migraineur, and some have speculated that his line drawings represented visual distortions experienced during his migraine auras. For today's medical authors, figures are an integral part of the writing.

Figures, also called illustrations, contain art and look more or less like a picture. This is a broad definition because figures include photographs and shaded drawings, line drawings, graphs, and algorithms. I prefer the term *figures* to *illustrations* because all are cited in the text using the word *Figure*, as shown below when I cite the figures in this chapter. Most medical review articles, research reports, and book chapters are enhanced by one or more graphs, drawings, algorithms, or photographs.

About Figures

One or more carefully selected and meticulously constructed illustrations can turn an average article into a great one. Some articles you decide to write will be clearly deficient without an illustration or two. For example, let's imagine that over the past year I have encountered three instances of sixth cranial nerve paralysis presenting as the initial manifestation of a pituitary tumor, and I wish to report these cases. Such a case report will be greatly enhanced by the addition of magnetic resonance images and perhaps by a photograph of one of the patients. One illustration may be just right and two or three too many. I need to see only one photo of a patient with ocular esotropia. Presenting illustrations showing the same physical finding in two more patients adds nothing.

Each figure must have a descriptive legend that allows the illustration to make sense on its own. As is true with tables, figures should not duplicate what is written in the text.

Displaying photographs or even drawings in which the person is recognizable presents special issues. Subjects must not be identifiable or their pictures must be accompanied by written permission for use. A parent or guardian's signature will be required for a child.[2]

Types of Figure

Halftones

This term applies to black and white photographs and also to drawings that include shades of gray. It also includes radiographic images. Halftones must be high quality, with good contrast. X-rays often lack good contrast, a problem that is magnified if the image must be reduced. Figure 4.1 combines a good-quality photograph and an x-ray that clearly shows the fracture.

Publishers generally prefer that figures be prepared as sharp, glossy black-and-white photographic prints, usually 127 × 173 mm (5 × 7 inches) but no larger than 203 × 254 mm (8 × 10 inches).[2] Letters and other symbols must be large enough to be read if and when the figure is reduced. Not all journals have the same requirements: the *Journal of Neurology* requests that all halftones "be trimmed at right angles and in the desired final size. Letters and numbers should be 3 mm high."[3]

Take good care of the artwork that you submit. You should never mark directly on a photographic print. Labels and

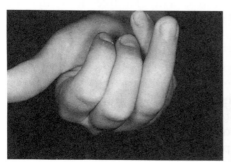
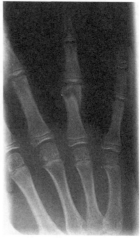

FIGURE 4.1.   High-quality halftones with good contrast showing the consequences of a fracture. (From Taylor RB. *Family medicine: principles and practice.* 6th ed. New York: Springer-Verlag, 2003, with permission.)

indicators should be submitted on an overlay, a duplicate print, or a photocopy of the original halftone.

Line Drawings

Sometimes line drawings can illustrate what you want to show better than a photograph. This is especially true in illustrating body anatomy. These drawings can sometimes be done by you and used directly in the article or book. Figure 4.2 is an illustration of a line drawing done by the author and included in a clinical reference book. In other instances you may draw a rough draft, which is then converted into the final artwork by a professional artist. Today it is customary to have medical illustrations prepared by a professional medical illustrator.

Working with a medical illustrator can be an art in itself. Sometimes you will hire the medical illustrator; at other times the publisher engages the illustrator. (In both instances, who pays the medical illustrator varies with the publication or, in the case of a book, with your contract.) When your art involves a professional, it is best to make personal contact

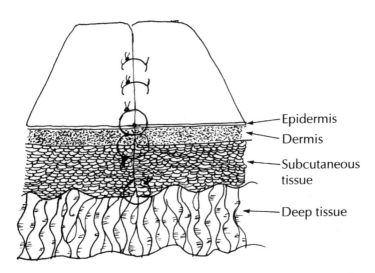

FIGURE 4.2.   A line drawing hand drawn by the author to illustrate a laceration repair. (From Taylor RB. *Family medicine: principles and practice.* 6th ed. New York: Springer-Verlag, 2003, with permission.)

and decide together how you will collaborate. In most instances, I have created my best effort, with labels, and given it to the medical illustrator to be made into professional-quality art. When doing so, you must be sure that your illustration is anatomically correct. If a vein is medial to an artery (as in the groin), then you must draw it so. Some medical illustrators know more anatomy than the average medical student; some do not. What is certain, however, is that it is expensive to alter completed line drawings.

The *New England Journal of Medicine* (NEJM) instructions for submission state: "Medical and scientific illustrations will be created or recreated in-house. Please submit a clear conceptual sketch of the figure and a comprehensive legend for the in-house illustrators to use as a reference.... If an outside illustrator creates the figure, the Journal reserves the right to modify or completely redraw it to meet our specifications for publication."[4]

When a professional medical illustrator creates art, there are special permission issues. The artist may prefer to approve "one-time use" only and wish to retain ownership rights to the figure. On the other hand, the journal or book publisher may not approve such an arrangement. In the instance of "outside" medical illustrators, the NEJM instructions to authors state: "The author must explicitly acquire all rights to the illustration from the artist in order for us to publish the illustration."[4]

A computer can be used to create some uncomplicated drawings. The *Journal of Neurology* states, "Computer drawings are acceptable provided they are of comparable quality to line drawings. Lines and curves must be smooth."[3] Figure 4.3 is an example of a line drawing created on computer.

Some simple drawings can be scanned into your electronic manuscript using a conventional office scanner, set at a minimum of 600 dpi (dots per inch). Drawings in shades of gray need 1200 dpi or greater, which may not be available on your office scanner.

Graphs

There are four basic types of graph: line graphs, bar charts, pie charts, and complex graphs. Line graphs are usually the

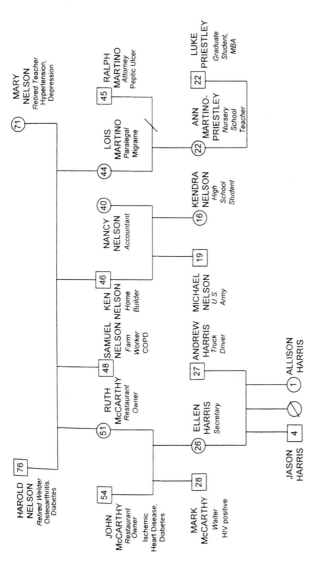

FIGURE 4.3. A line drawing created on computer showing a family genogram. (From Taylor RB. *Family medicine: principles and practice.* 6th ed. New York: Springer-Verlag, 2003, with permission.)

Nelson family genogram: family members, occupations, chronic health problems. Symbols used: ☐, male, age 76; ◯, female, age 71; ☐○, marriage; ☐/○, divorce; ∅, deceased.

best choice when showing what happens over time (Fig. 4.4). A bar chart can also show trends over time, or it can be used to compare relative amounts such as the incomes or work hours of various medical specialties. Choose a pie chart to show proportions such as how many of your clinic's patients have private insurance, Medicare, Medicaid, or no insurance at all. Complex charts may be scatter diagrams or combine lines, bars, or even pie drawings.

Sometimes data can best be shown graphically, and computers have made graph creation quite easy. Various software options are available and can sometimes be as simple as the Microsoft Excel program on your computer.

Various publications have different requirements for graphs and charts. JAMA requires high-quality resolution (600 dpi).[1] NEJM requests "1200 dpi/ppi for black and white line art. This refers to strictly black-and-white images such as line graphs."[4]

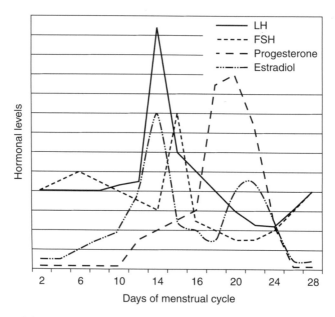

Figure 4.4. A line graph that illustrates hormone changes through the menstrual cycle. (From Taylor RB. *Family medicine: principles and practice.* 6th ed. New York: Springer-Verlag, 2003, with permission.)

Algorithms

Algorithms are combinations of graph and table. The word *algorithm* comes from the name of a 9th century Arabic mathematician, al-Khowarizmi. The algorithm is an excellent way to show a decision tree, as shown in Figure 4.5. I like to use

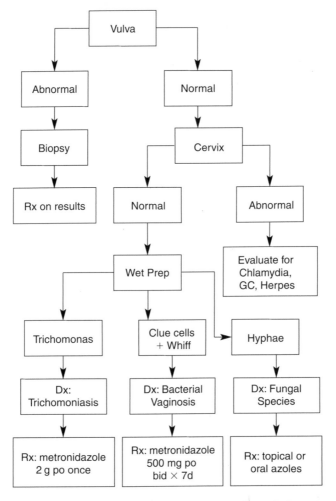

Figure 4.5. An algorithm that illustrates a decision tree for vaginal symptoms. (From Taylor RB. *Family medicine: principles and practice.* 6th ed. New York: Springer-Verlag, 2003, with permission.)

an algorithm to illustrate specific steps in clinical reasoning: If the patient has this symptom, do this and not that. If there is this physical sign, obtain this laboratory test, but that one is not needed.

On the negative side, I find algorithms difficult to construct both medically and technically. On the medical side, decisions often depend on more than one variable, and the algorithm may not allow presentation of all the possible influences on a diagnostic or therapeutic choice. Technically, algorithms generally call for diagonal lines or even lines that bend around boxes; I find these difficult to draw on a computer, and if not submitted in camera-ready copy, errors can occur in production.

In the end, I use algorithms when it is clearly the best way to present a decision tree. Otherwise I prefer figures that are easier to create and to comprehend.

Submitting Figures with Your Manuscript

Every figure must have a legend (just as every table must have a title) that fully describes what is presented. JAMA sets a limit of 40 words.[1] If submitting hardcopy, type the legend double-spaced on a separate sheet of paper and submit it at the end of the manuscript. Do not position the legend in the figure itself; legend and figure are handled separately in production.

As with tables, camera-ready copy is usually the best way to submit your figures. It may cost more to obtain the photographic images, but publishers like such submissions and you will see fewer errors in print. On the back of each figure, affix a label with the figure number, short title of the figure, your name, short title of the manuscript, and an arrow indicating the top of the figure. Do not write directly on the back of the figure, especially on the back of photographs. I have seen more than one photograph ruined by writing on the reverse side.

If you have questions about submitting your favorite PowerPoint slides or using Adobe Illustrator or other programs, call the journal's editorial office.

How many "original" copies of photographs and other art must be sent when the journal requests three or four copies of the manuscript with original submission? The ideal would be to send publication-quality copies of all illustrations with each copy of the manuscript. If this is not possible, be sure to send one publication copy and copies of figures that are of sufficient quality for review. For hardcopy submissions, JAMA requests "one set of figures and three sets of copies. For black-and-white graphs and illustrations, provide high-resolution (600 dpi minimum) laser printouts."[1]

COPYRIGHT

Do not worry too much about copyright. The law and the ethics of medical publishing protect us quite well.

Copyright is a form of protection provided by United States law to authors of "original works of authorship," including literary, dramatic, musical, artistic, and certain other intellectual works. Section 106 of the 1976 Copyright Act generally gives the owner of copyright the exclusive right to do and to authorize others to do the following:

- Reproduce the work in copies or phonorecords;
- Prepare derivative works based on the work;
- Perform the work publicly in the case of performance art; and
- Display the copyrighted work publicly.[5]

The Copyright Act holds that protection begins "when the pen leaves the keyboard." This means that you hold copyright to your article immediately upon creation of the work. The intellectual property rights of the author are separate from the publication of the work.

There is at least one important exception to the "author holds the copyright" principle: the "work made for hire." This includes a work prepared by an employee within the scope of employment and a work ordered or commissioned, such as an instructional text or a translation. There may or may not be a written agreement that a work is considered a work made for hire.[5]

In fact, with a work made for hire or, for that matter, with any medical article or book, copyright rarely becomes an issue. This is true because medical publishers insist that copyright be assigned to them, in writing, as a condition of publishing the work. That means that of all the books and articles I have published, I currently own the copyrights to only a few of them. The few exceptions are old books that are out of print and the publishers have returned all rights to me as a courtesy.

In all other instances, the publisher holds the copyright. As I type these words, I own the copyright to them; by the time you read this, the publisher, Springer-Verlag, New York, will hold copyright.

What is the significance of not owning the copyright to my works? Not much. I can think of two items to mention. One is that I must seek permission from Springer-Verlag Publishers if I wish to use big chunks of text, tables, or figures from my Springer-Verlag books in writing for any other publisher. Getting such permission involves sending a request (see below), and has not been a large problem. The second time copyright ownership comes to my attention is when other authors request permission to use something published in my books. The publisher now charges a fee for this permission and shares the revenue with me; on each royalty statement I find a (very small) payment for "permissions granted."

Inexperienced authors sometime wonder whether someone will steal their great idea if they submit a proposal to a journal or book publisher. I am happy to report that medical editors have much higher moral standards than many chief executive officers of large corporations. Also, there really are very few article or book ideas that are revolutionary and worth pilfering. You are quite safe in sending proposals and article ideas.

BORROWED MATERIALS AND PERMISSIONS

I wrote above that you should not worry excessively about copyright. In contrast, you should be concerned about permissions if you intend to borrow words, tables, art, or anything else from previously published work, even your own. In Chapter 5, I discuss plagiarism. Here I discuss the situations in which you need permission to use borrowed material and how to get the documents you need.

Let's first look at what's free: All government publications may be used without seeking permission. For example, in the previous section I listed the rights protected by the 1976 Copyright Act. What appears on the page is almost word for word what is on the U.S. Copyright Office Web site. I did not use quotations around the material because I edited out some discussion about sound recording, pantomimes, and choreographic work, which we rarely encounter in medical writing. I did, however, give attribution by citing the Web site, because that allows the reader to seek more in-depth information and because it is the ethical thing to do. However, if I had not attributed the words by citing the U.S. Copyright Office as the source, I would have technically be within my legal rights.

When Do I Need to Seek Permission for Use of Borrowed Material?

Part of the answer is easy. You need permission to reproduce any previously published table or figure. You also need permission to "adapt" any table or figure. If you use data from four studies to create your own table or figure, I think that the creation is yours and no permission is needed; you must identify your data sources in the table or figure legend. Some editors may disagree with my opinion about tables or figures based on multiple published studies and will require that you seek permissions from all sources.

The next gray issue is the use of text (phrases, sentences, and paragraphs) from published sources. All borrowed work, even a few words, should be attributed to the source. This may be done in a number of ways, cited in the text as I did with the Pogo quotation in a previous chapter or as a formal reference. This protects you from allegations of plagiarism. You borrowed the words and told where you got them.

What about a few sentences or more? When do you need to seek permission for use? This is murky, and the answer is not nearly as clear as with tables and figures. The doctrine involves "fair use" and you will see allusions to needing permission to borrow *lengthy quotations*. What constitutes "fair use" and how long is a "lengthy quotation?" It is very, very rarely that a legal issue arises. I can think of no examples. Allegations of plagiarism are one thing; legal complaints are quite unlikely when the author has borrowed a quotation with careful attribution to the source. I don't think anyone has given a definition of *fair use* and *lengthy quotation*, since all legal issues are ultimately settled by trial or mutual agreement. Court decisions have described fair use as including "short passages of a scholarly or technical work, for illustration or clarification of the author's observations."[6] I will go out on a limb and state that you should seek permission if you are quoting more than 100 words, even with attribution.

Who Must I Contact to Obtain Permission?

The answer to this question is also not always clear. I always start with the publisher, and I include in my letter (Fig. 4.6) a question about anyone else that must be contacted. Since publishers always hold copyright to published articles and books, their permission for borrowed use should be sufficient. Nevertheless some permissions editors (yes, such persons exist) insist that you also seek permission from authors; some do not.

One special problem may be medical illustrations created by an artist hired by the author. The artist may have successfully contracted with the author and publisher for "one-time" use of the figure you wish to use. In this instance, you will need to track down the artist, an often difficult journey, and obtain written permission. You will also almost certainly be asked to pay a fee.

Who Is Responsible for Getting Permissions?

The answer is short and direct: You are. The author is responsible for getting acceptable permissions and submitting them with the manuscript. I have reprinted in this book two borrowed illustrations (from the same journal). I sent a request for permission as soon as the book contract was signed, long before I began working on the chapter containing the figures.

There is one very good reason to seek permissions early. The article or book cannot be published until all permissions have been submitted and approved. When you consider the

---

Letterhead

Date:

Dear:

In the forthcoming book, **The Clinician's Guide to Medical Writing**, to be published by Springer-Verlag – New York Publishers, I request permission to reprint the following material:

Author(s):

Book/Journal/Article Title:

Specific Material:

I request your permission to reprint the material specified, with nonexclusive world rights in the forthcoming book and all future editions, translations and revisions, including electronic media. If you agree, please indicate by signing and returning this letter. Full credit will be given to the author and publisher. If you do not control these rights in their entirety, please let me know with whom I should communicate and kindly provide me with an address.

Consideration of this request at your earliest convenience will be greatly appreciated.

Thank you,

Robert B. Taylor, MD

Please return to:

> Robert B. Taylor, MD
> Oregon Health & Science University, Mail Code FM
> 3181 SW Sam Jackson Park Road
> Portland, Oregon 97239-3098

....

We grant the permission requested on the terms stated in this letter

By: ....   Date: ....

FIGURE 4.6.   Sample permission letter. This letter should be modified by substituting your article or book name, identifying the requested material, and adding your name as the requester. Then print on your own letterhead.

difficulty you may encounter in finding the person or persons who can actually sign your form, it pays to get moving on this task.

One of the surprises in medical writing may be the cost of permissions and the length of some of the forms that must be completed. A typical fee is $50 per table or figure used. The online permission request form of the American Psychiatric Association that applies to works in their journals and books is two pages long. Be prepared.

How Do I Obtain Permission?

Find the address of the publisher and send the form. Publisher addresses can almost always be found in a Google search, as described in Chapter 1. Also, you should be taking your quotation, table, or figure directly from the original journal or book, and most of these publications contain a valid mailing address.

In my experience, no publisher has ever questioned my standard permission request, as shown in Figure 4.6, although some have qualified their responses.

My chief problem arises when publishers qualify their response. Favorite replies are stamped on my letter, telling me that the permission for use is "valid for only one edition of the book," "not to include electronic media," or "for English-language publication only." I wish publishers would not do this, especially when they are charging me. But they do. If any of these issues are important to you, I think you need to contact the permissions editor and ask what needs to be done.

I hope that all the above has persuaded you to create your own tables and figures whenever possible. It is usually easier than getting (and paying for) permission, and you have added something new to the medical literature.

REFERENCE CITATIONS

Virtually all medical writing contains references, and although each publication has its own reference style, most follow the method of the International Committee of Medical Journal Editors (ICMJE). In fact, the instructions for JAMA, NEJM and ICMJE all differ very slightly, notably in how they

TABLE 4.2.   Examples of the three most common types of references

---

Article citation: if six authors or fewer list all; if seven or more authors list the first three and then add "et al"):
1. Corey L, Wald A, Patel R, et al. Once-daily valacyclovir to reduce the risk of transmission of genital herpes. N Engl J Med 2004;350:11–20.

Book citation, noting chapter and authors:
2. Arevalo JA, Nesbitt TS. Medical problems during pregnancy. In: Taylor RB, editor. Family medicine: principles and practice. 6th ed. New York: Springer-Verlag; 2003:109–116.

Electronic source:
3. Journal of the American Medical Association. Instructions for authors. Available at: http://jama.ama-assn.org/ifora_current/dtl. Accessed 12 Dec 2004.

---

choose to cite books as sources. Do not worry about this. The differences are minor, usually regarding punctuation. The information needed is the same for all and, if your style is not exactly what the journal uses, the copyeditor will make the small changes in periods, commas and semicolons. In my opinion, this issue will not cause rejection of a good paper. Table 4.2 lists examples of the three most common types of citations. I suggest that you copy this table and tape it to your computer.

Number references in the order that they appear in the text. Do not alphabetize your reference list unless this is the style of your journal. Citation numbers in the text should follow the journal's style, which may be superscript or in parentheses. Unless you are attempting to submit a camera-ready article, the way you present your text citations, just like how you punctuate your reference list, is not a deal-breaker. Just be sure all the information is included and is presented clearly and consistently.

Verify all references against the original sources. Do not "borrow" from someone else's list of citations. It is perfectly permissible to use a published list as source for your research, just as you would use PubMed. But then you must seek out and read the original publication.

Verification also includes reading the cited sources carefully to be sure that the source says what you think it does. If you do not do this, someone knowledgeable in the field will surely spot the "cognitive dissonance," and correct you in a letter to the editor.

When you are finished with the paper, keep all your reference files, which are likely to be useful in future writing.

ACKNOWLEDGMENT

Figures 4.1 to 4.5 are from Taylor RB. Family medicine: principles and practice. 6th ed. New York: Springer-Verlag, 2003. I am indebted to the contributing authors who created these figures.

REFERENCES

1. Journal of the American Medical Association. Instructions for authors. JAMA 2004:291:125–131. Available at: http://jama. ama-assn.org/ifora_current/dtl.
2. International Committee of Medical Journal Editors. Uniform requirements for manuscripts submitted to biomedical journals. Updated October 2001. http://www.icmje.org.
3. Journal of Neurology. Instructions to authors. Available at: http://www.springerlink.com.
4. New England Journal of Medicine. Instructions for submission—help for authors. Available at: http://www.nejm.org/hfa/techfig.asp.
5. U.S. Copyright Office. Copyright basics (Circular 1). Available at: http://www.copyright.gov/circs/circ1.html.
6. Keyt Law: Business, Internet, e-commerce, and domain name law. Available at: http://www.keytlaw.com/Copyrights/fairuse.htm.

5

What's Special About Medical Writing?

Frey[1] states, "Writing is a historical act. The role of written communication has been to document human history; our knowledge of human culture and values exist because some-one has written about it." There is also writing that is lost, or has not been deciphered yet. We know little about early central African cultures because no one recorded what happened at the time. Our knowledge of Mayan and Inca cultures is defi-cient because most of their writing was destroyed by zealous Christians. Native American languages were first written in 1921, when a phonetic alphabet of 86 symbols was developed by a Cherokee named Sequoyah; this feat was honored when the redwood tree was named *Sequoia*.[2] It was 1952 when we began to decipher the written language of ancient Crete.[3]

In the sciences, writing records the evolution of ideas. In the middle ages, influenza was considered to be caused by celestial "influence," although we now know that the cause is a virus. We once treated a variety of illnesses by bleeding the patient; now this therapy is reserved for the management of polycythemia. One of the joys of writing over a lifetime is to read your own past published works, just to see how pre-scient (or how wrong) you were.

Poetry, short stories, mystery novels, historical documents, and other types of writing all have their peculiarities and conventions. Medical writing is, first of all, factual. It is expository. Opinions must be clearly stated as such. Values are typically implied, rather than stated. The chief virtue is knowledge, especially new knowledge.

In a sense, the peculiarities of medical writing are what make it special: These include the imperative that what is printed is as true as current knowledge allows. We strive to state things correctly and precisely. We should avoid jargon, be accurate in what we say, and be careful with abbreviations and acronyms. In addition, in contrast to our colleagues who write fiction, there is the tendency of medical authors to write as groups. Finally, we clinician-writers face a minefield of ethical issues that can impair our credibility or worse.

ABOUT MEDICAL JOURNALS

Types of Journals

Medical journals are not all alike. Although many journals do not fit into the categorization I am about to use, I think of medical journals in a hierarchy consisting of four types. I hope you see the merits of this hierarchy; you will certainly see its lack of specificity.

Broad-Based Peer-Reviewed Journal

A peer-reviewed journal is defined by the International Committee of Medical Journal Editors (ICMJE)[4] as "one that has submitted most of its published articles for review by experts who are not part of the editorial staff." These journals are at the top of the scholarly food chain. Most of their content is composed of reports of original research. They contain advertising, but also have a large base of paid subscriber support.

Many hold that there are a "big four" of peer-reviewed journals that are read and respected internationally: the *New England Journal of Medicine* (NEJM), *The Lancet*, the *British Medical Journal* (BMJ), and the *Journal of the American Medical Association* (JAMA). For example, the *British Medical Journal*, published by the BMJ Publishing Group, "aims to publish rigorous, accessible and entertaining material that will help doctors and medical students in their daily practice, lifelong learning and career development." The BMJ has a weekly circulation of more than 100,000. The NEJM is published by the Massachusetts Medical Society, although its circulation far exceeds the number of physicians in the state. *Lancet* is published weekly by Elsevier Publishers and can be accessed on line at http://www.thelancet.com. JAMA is published by the American Medical Association and members receive the journal as a membership benefit; many non-AMA members subscribe.

Most of the more than 4000 scientific and medical journals published in the world are peer reviewed. Few have strong support from paid subscribers.

Specialty Oriented Peer-Reviewed Journals

Because it pulls no punches in its name, *Gut* is one of my favorite journal names. It is the official journal of the British Society of Gastroenterology, and is edited by the BMJ journals department. Membership in the Aerospace Medical Association includes a subscription to the peer-reviewed monthly journal, *Aviation, Space, and Environmental Medicine*. The *American Journal of Surgery*, published by Elsevier Publishers, is the official publication for six different surgical societies.

Some of these publications are owned by specialty organizations and are heavily subsidized by dues. Others are more dependent on advertiser support.

Not all of these journals publish reports of original research. *American Family Physician*, published by the American Academy of Family Physicians, publishes peer-reviewed review articles and virtually no original research. Its total circulation exceeds 190,000.

Controlled-Circulation Journals

These publications are entirely dependent on advertising for survival. They are sometimes called "throw-aways," but I have always considered the epithet to be unfair and elitist. The truth is that practicing physicians read journals such as *Postgraduate Medicine*, *Consultant*, and *Medical Economics*. Years ago, I had the experience of publishing an article, "How to See Office Patients More Efficiently" in one of these journals, *Physicians' Management*, and in the same month I published a scholarly article in a peer-reviewed research journal. Several of my practicing colleagues congratulated me on the practice-based article; none mentioned the research report.

Most of the controlled-circulation publications specialize in some way. There is *The Female Patient*, with review articles about health problems of women; *Cutis*, covering diseases of the skin; and *Hospital Practice*, presenting topics related to inpatient care.

Online Journals

Hospitalist is an online journal for those who specialize in inpatient care. Its Web site looks much like a printed journal. It has an index, an editor's page, articles, editorials, and even a "job opportunity" listing. At this time, *Hospitalist* does not seem to be peer-reviewed. On balance, it receives no funding from a pharmaceutical company, medical organization, or insurance company.

The Public Library of Science plans to offer a free online journal that makes research reports free to anyone who logs onto its Web site.

At this time, I place online journals at the bottom of the hierarchy. This may change. Free and fast access to information is the future of medical communication. In the next edition of this book, my hierarchy may look different.

Indexing and the Impact Factor

Some medical journals are "indexed" and some are not; those that are not would like to be. A medical journal such as *Gut* can be—and is—"indexed" in one of three ways: Index Medicus, the Excerpta Medica Database (EMBASE), and the Institute for Scientific Information (ISI). What does this all mean, and why might it be important for the medical writer?

Briefly stated, indexing means that the publications in a journal are listed in one of the three databases noted above. Publishing your article in an indexed journal means that when an author or a scientist consults PubMed or another reference site on your topic, your article will appear on the list. Without indexing, your article is not found by others and, although brilliant and ground-breaking, it may languish in obscurity.

Note that whether or not your article is indexed is determined not by the excellence of your article, but by where it is published. Each of the index organizations makes ongoing decisions as to which journals are indexed and which requests are denied. Index Medicus/MEDLINE makes its decisions based on:

Scientific merit of a journal's content: validity, importance, originality, and contribution to the field

The objectivity, credibility, and quality of its contents
Production quality
An audience of health professionals
Types of content, consisting of one or more of:
  Reports of original research
  Original clinical observations with analysis
  Analysis of philosophical, ethical, or social aspects of
  medicine
  Critical reviews
  Statistical compilations
  Descriptions or evaluations of methods or procedures
  Case reports with discussions

Note that the report of original research is not the only type of article included in Index Medicus. Review article journals may be accepted.

The Three Index Databases

Index Medicus and its online counterpart, MEDLINE, are used internationally to provide access to the world's biomedical literature. Both are part of the National Library of Medicine. *Index Medicus* currently contains more than 4000 titles. For more information, go to: http://www.nlm.nih.gov/tsd/serials/lji.html.

EMBASE, the *Excerpta Medica* database, is a biomedical and pharmaceutical database that gives information to medical and drug-related subjects. EMBASE contains approximately 9 million items, with 450,000 added annually. It is especially good for drug-related searches. Access EMBASE at: http://www.embase.com.

The *Institute for Scientific Information*, a business of the Thompson Corporation, publishes *Journal Citation Reports* (JCR) and the *Science Citations Index*. The ISI *Web of Science* is a multidisciplinary collection of bibliographic information from more than 8600 scholarly journals.

The Journal Impact Factor

In the 1960s, ISI developed the journal "impact factor." What is the impact factor and how does it relate to my favorite journals? First proposed by Garfield,[5] the impact factor is a method of rating the influence of a journal and comparing this numerically to a large number of other journals. It does so by measuring the number of citations to articles published in a journal averaged over two years; then this number is divided by the total number of articles published in the journal over the same period. Table 5.1 lists the impact factor for some selected journals; the higher the number, the greater the presumed "impact" of the journal.

Just for interest, the five top-rated journals and their impact factors for 2001 were:[6]

Annual Review of Immunology (50.340)
Annual Review of Biochemistry (43.429)
Cell (32.440)
New England Journal of Medicine (29.512)
Nature Medicine (27.905)

As might be expected, some researchers are critical of the impact factor. Ojasoo et al[7] observe: "The choice of citations is subjective and the non-pertinence of the citations is well known. Several variables may intervene, such as the type of journal and its size, domain concerned, language of the publication, self-citations, coding of the articles depending on their nature, and the choice of the manuscripts published ('hot papers')." The impact factor is an indicator of citation numbers and not of their quality, and can certainly not be used to assess an author's work.[7]

TABLE 5.1. Impact factors of selected journals

Journal	Impact factor
Annals of Internal Medicine	10.097
British Medical Journal	5.143
Journal of General Internal Medicine	2.067
Journal of the American Medical Association	11.435
Medical Journal of Australia	1.973
Preventive Medicine	1.631

Data from http://www.infomed.sld.cu/instituciones/ipk/biblioweb/impact_factor.htm.

Some journals post their current impact factor on their Web sites. At www.nature.com/nm/, the home page of *Nature Medicine* states that its latest available (2002) impact factor is 28.740. In an ideal world, your article will be published in the journal with the highest possible impact factor, but without making a special effort you may never learn the number and its comparators. Although the impact factor is seldom of great importance to the beginning medical writer, you will encounter the term and should know what it means. I will return to the impact factor in Chapter 10, when I discuss getting your work in print.

How Clinicians Read Medical Journals

As a medical writer, you should pause to consider how clinicians read the medical literature. Do clinicians read each journal cover to cover, beginning with page one, studying all sections of each article? No, they don't. In practice, I propose three ways in which clinicians read journals: They graze, hunt, and gorge.[8]

Grazing

Clinicians are most likely to *graze* the paper journals that cross their desk, and they do so when they have "spare time." There are just too many publications to read each in depth. For example, I receive JAMA and NEJM each week, several monthly journals in my specialty, and about six or eight controlled circulation publications. The only way to handle the volume is to *graze*. By this I mean that I read the table of contents carefully. If I see a title that looks interesting, I will turn to the first page of the article and read the abstract. If I am very interested in the method and results of the study, I will read those sections and the summary. I estimate that I read the abstracts of every fourth or fifth article, and then I read about one fourth of these in depth.

In fact, several journals include a synopsis of major articles. One of these is the NEJM, which publishes "This Week in the Journal," a section early in each weekly issue that presents a brief synopsis of each major article. JAMA summarizes the issue's articles in "This Week in JAMA." These short summaries may be all that many busy clinicians read.

The grazing habits of readers have implications for medical writers: First, compose your title with great care, because this is likely to be the only part of the article read by up to 90% of your intended audience. Then, devote the same care to the abstract; of those who turn to your article, up to 75% of readers will stop here. Of course, I tend to pay more attention to my two "major" journals—JAMA and the NEJM—and to the leading journal in my specialty. This means that less prestigious publications get less attention.

Do I have data to support the grazing numbers above? Not really. I can state that what I describe is how I read journals. I did a literature search when I wrote the editorial cited in reference 8, and found a small, diverse, and largely unhelpful group of studies on how we clinicians read the medical literature. If your reading habits are different, I would be pleased to hear from you.

Hunting

When clinicians need information about a specific problem, we *hunt* for answers. Years ago, I would hunt in my file of journal clippings or go to the library. Now hunting is done online. Seldom do I go to a paper journal to hunt for a clinical fact. My file of journal clippings is becoming a historical curiosity.

The tendency to hunt makes it vital that your important studies are published in indexed journals. Those who read your work are likely never to hold the actual journal in their hands; but by locating your work online and citing it in future scientific articles, these writers disseminate your findings and advance medical knowledge.

Gorging

We writers would like to think that each reader ponders every word we write. To do so would be to *gorge*—to take in way too much. Perhaps the most sedentary, semiretired emeritus professor has the luxury of reading every word of every article in every journal.

GETTING IT RIGHT

In a speech in the United States Senate in 1850, Henry Clay stated, "I would rather be right than be president." I hope that he was right, because he never became president.

For the medical writer, being "right" is paramount. More than probably any other discipline, medical science is unforgiving about errors. The requirement to present truthful information is one of the special aspects of medical writing. Your data must be factual, your conclusions justified, your recommendations based on evidence, your opinions unbiased, and your writing "right."

Medical Jargon

We clinicians love medical jargon: We turn nouns into verbs, such as "to scope" or "to surgerize" a patient. We use cute phrases such as the patient having "antibiotic deficiency." We "turf" a patient when making a transfer of care. Not surprisingly, much medical jargon originates with young clinicians, sometimes sleep-deprived, as they busily care for patients. The terms are often shorthand, sometimes intended to speak to one another in code without the patient understanding ("lues" used to refer to syphilis, for example), and may be derogatory (GOMER, see page 117).

Jordan and Shepard[9] propose a nicely written definition of jargon: "Jargon refers to technical expressions used by a profession or cult which by no stretch of the imagination can be considered good English and which are often confusing, not only to those outside the fold, but often also to those within it." Table 5.2 lists some examples of medical jargon.

Accuracy and Precision

When I am frantically searching for the treatment of a disease, it helps me little to read that the patient should receive, "a first- or second-generation cephalosporin, 250–500 mg every 8 to 12 hours." It is even more frustrating if a drug is mentioned without a recommended dose. Worst of all, by far, would be a wrong dose.

TABLE 5.2. Medical jargon: some selected examples

Jargon word or phrase	What you probably mean to say
Digitalize	To initiate therapy with a digitalis derivative; or perhaps to perform a digital rectal examination
Diabetic	A patient who has diabetes mellitus
Prepped	Prepared for surgery
Acute abdomen	Acute condition of the abdomen, often requiring surgery
Negative	Absence of abnormalities
Gland	Lymph node
To appendectomize	To perform an appendectomy
To buff a chart	To be sure the medical record is complete and accurate
Antibiotic deficiency	Indicating that the patient has an infection that warrants antibiotic use
To turf (a patient)	The act of referring a patient to another clinician or institution
FLK	A term that clinicians really should not use, meaning "funny-looking kid"

In my files is an Errata Notice, received from a major medical publisher and referring to what was a newly published major medical reference book. Happily I was not the author or editor of the potentially fatal error that prompted the following notice:

> Table 116–1 on page 880 and the bottom line in the left-hand column on page 881 erroneously indicate that the dilution of epinephrine to be used for intracardiac injection in cases of cardiac arrest is 1:1000. The correct dilution is *1:10,000.*

"Reading maketh a full man; conference a ready man; and writing an exact man," wrote Francis Bacon (1561–1626). The value of months of research and writing can be undermined by a single factual error in a published paper. If you have published a book with an error, a reviewer will unfailingly discover this mistake and report to the world when writing the critical review. In the many stages between your keystroke and the printed page—copyediting, typesetting, and correcting proofs—there are ample opportunities for errors. The careful author will pay close attention at each stage.

What are common sources of errors and how can they be avoided? If writing a report of research, double-check all data, especially your statistical analysis. Scrutinize all numerical data, especially—as noted above—drug doses. As mentioned in Chapter 4, pay special attention to tables and figures. Be sure any headings are correct. Check all references against original sources to verify that each citation is correct and that the referenced source supports what you say it does in your text. Each page, each paragraph, each sentence, and each word must be examined by asking, "Is there some error that I am overlooking?"

Abbreviations and Acronyms as Sometimes Misleading Shortcuts

Among the items that can cloud meaning and introduce errors are abbreviations and acronyms (AA).

Abbreviations

As a reader, I wish that writers would use fewer abbreviations. The rule is that you can create any abbreviation you wish as long as you identify it with first use. For example, I created an abbreviation for the phrase used in the previous, *abbreviations and acronyms*. From now on in this chapter I am free to use either the phrase or the abbreviation. The problem is that I may not use the abbreviation for another six pages, and the reader using this book as a reference source and encountering this abbreviation later on must search this entire chapter to discover that, on these pages, AA does not mean Alcoholics Anonymous.

Here are some of my guidelines for the use of abbreviations:

■ Don't use more than one abbreviation in a sentence. Think twice if you are tempted to write something like, "The patient who has IUGR or PPROM has an increased risk of PTL and PTB." (Translation for those who don't do maternity care: The patient who has intrauterine growth retardation or pre-term premature rupture of the membranes has an increased risk of pre-term labor and pre-term birth.)

■ Do not use an abbreviation in an article title. Sure, there will be exceptions such as "... prevalence in the U.S." However, generally you should spell out all words in the title. Remember that you should explain an abbreviation with first use, and the title is not the place to do this.

■ Try to avoid abbreviations in the abstract. Here it will be possible to explain the abbreviation, but since most of your readers won't read the body of your paper anyhow, why break the flow by stating your abbreviation meaning here?

■ Be careful of "standard" abbreviations. What is standard today can change. Do you remember when "mg%" was the standard?

When properly selected, abbreviations can be a space-saving convenience. If used improperly, they can introduce confusion. Table 5.3 lists some examples of abbreviations that can be misunderstood. In addition, I have included in Appendix 3 a handy list of commonly used abbreviations.

TABLE 5.3. Examples of abbreviations that may mislead readers

Abbreviation	What the abbreviation might mean
BP	This abbreviation means blood pressure, doesn't it? Not always. BP may also indicate bedpan, bathroom privileges, bullous pemphigoid, or even British Pharmacopoeia.
DI	When you see DI, think of diabetes insipidus—or perhaps diagnostic imaging, detrusor instability, drug interaction, or date of injury.
ID	When you see this abbreviation, choose from among identification, infectious disease, intradermal, or initial dose.
IT	Possibilities include intensive therapy, inhalation therapy, or even incentive therapy. Confusion between intrathecal and intratracheal when administering medication could be harmful.
MI	MI might mean myocardial infarction or mitral insufficiency.
ROM	This might stand for range of motion, right otitis media, or rupture of membranes.
TD	Think of test dose, tardive dyskinesia, transverse diameter, tetanus-diphtheria toxoid, temporary disability, or traveler's diarrhea. But, in a medical setting, not *touchdown*.

Acronyms

These are words made up of initial letters or syllables or a group of words. An acronym usually is typed in all capital letters. SCUBA is an acronym for "self-contained underwater breathing apparatus." Writing scuba or Scuba is incorrect. World War II gave us a rich trove of acronyms: AWOL (Absent WithOut Leave), SONAR (SOund NAvigation Ranging), and CINCUS (Commander In Chief of the United States Navy).

We pronounce the acronym as a word; CINCUS was pronounced, "Sink us." TURP, representing transurethral resection of the prostate, is pronounced "turp," rhyming with "burp." Abbreviations are pronounced letter by letter; human immunodeficiency virus infection is pronounced "H-I-V," sounding out all the letters. But acquired immunodeficiency syndrome has become the acronym AIDS. Some day we may, in fact, have forgotten what the four letters once stood for, just as most persons today know of SONAR, but don't recall the origin of the word.

Here are some examples of medical acronyms:

- ACE inhibitors: angiotensin-converting enzyme inhibitors are used to treat hypertension and other illnesses.
- CABG: pronounced "cabbage," the acronym stands for coronary artery bypass graft.
- CREST syndrome: a cluster of limited scleroderma skin manifestations and late visceral involvement that includes calcinosis, Raynaud's phenomenon, esophageal dysmotility, sclerodactyly, and telangiectasia.
- ELISA: with the enzyme-linked immunosorbent assay, the addition of "test" is redundant.
- GOMER: from "Get Outta My Emergency Room." The somewhat cynical author Shem describes the GOMER as "a human being who has lost—often through age—what goes into being a human being."[10]
- HIPPA: currently on the minds of clinicians, this acronym stands for the Health Insurance Portability and Accountability Act of 1996. HIPPA has become a splendid example of the law of unintended consequences.
- RICE: rest, ice, compression, and elevation are all used to treat acute injuries.

WRITING AS A TEAM SPORT

Medical writing is often done in teams. In research, teams are important because various people can bring different abilities: expertise in research methods, access to subjects, grant-writing experience, personal contacts in grant funding sources, and statistical skills. Writing groups may be clinicians with similar abilities and experience, or may include the young person with ambition and energy, the mid-level professional who knows how to get the job done, and the senior person whose participation helps assure eventual publication.

Writing as a team has other advantages: If I have a good writing or research idea and share it with others on a team, at a later time one of them is likely to have his or her own good idea and I will be included. In this way we all gain writing experience and entries on our curriculum vitae (CV). And, very important, our publication successes help advance medical knowledge and understanding.

Working as part of a team can help get the job done in a practical way. When everyone on the team has a task vital to the success of the project, no one is going to want to let the group down. In my college sociology class, the professor called this a "group effect." It certainly helps keep the writing project moving.

Guidelines for the Writing Team

Every writing team has implicit rules for how each person will act. Some groups have more explicit rules. The following are my suggested guidelines for the writing team:

- Decide upon a leader. The leader is usually the one with the "good idea" and the one who calls the meetings. The person who leads need not be the most senior person, but the leader must have a strong commitment to the project.
- Commit to regular meetings of the writing team. These meetings may be monthly or every 2 weeks. The frequency is not as important as the fact that they are on everyone's schedule. Also, all team members must show up. If someone misses several meetings, someone in the group must question that person's commitment to the project.

■ Decide on the role of each member of the team. The key person is the one who will lead the writing. In most cases, this person will compose the first draft, based on contributions from all. Then all team members will submit revision suggestions. In an efficient team, the lead writer has discretion to accept or reject revision suggestions.

■ Establish deadlines and then stick to them. Breaking any writing project into achievable deadlines makes it seem much more manageable. An example of deadlines for a review article might look something like:

Data collected by end of month 1

Outline completed by the end of month 2

First draft completed by the end of month 3

Second draft completed by end of month 4

Third revised draft completed by end of month 5

Final draft completed and in the mail in month 6

■ Decide early on the order of authorship. The person who has done most of the writing should usually be the first author, but not always.

Why Problems Develop in Writing Teams

Problems can develop in writing teams for a number of reasons:

■ Failure of leadership. In this instance, the leader is not leading. This person may be the one who calls the meetings and coordinates the task, but not the person doing the bulk of the writing. In this role, leading means taking charge, assigning roles, setting agendas and keeping the group moving.

■ Disagreements about how authors will be listed. Many teams dissolve in anger over this issue.

■ There is a slacker in the group. Someone is not getting the job done, and the problem is especially onerous if the slacker has a key job, such as getting funding or performing statistical analysis. When this occurs, members of the writing team need an "intervention," with a gentle, but firm confrontation.

■ Group wordsmithing. Wordsmithing by two people is tedious. Attempting wordsmithing by more than two people can be like fingernails on a chalkboard. Wordsmithing is and should be a solitary activity, based on written, repeat *written*, suggestions from others on the team.

■ The power play. Someone in the group is exerting undue force. The power play may be a challenge to the leader, or it might be an attempted veto: "I won't let this paper be submitted with my name on it unless this sentence is omitted." When this happens, the leader must make decisions, and the whole team must be involved.

Who on the Team Is an Author?

The issue of authorship on the final paper should be discussed in an early meeting. Every person whose name is listed at the top of a paper as author should qualify for authorship. And, on the other side of the coin, everyone who contributed substantially to the paper should be listed (see Ghost Authors, below). Each listed author should be ready to assume professional responsibility for some portion of the work.[11] In Chapter 9, I present more details about this important issue.

ETHICAL ISSUES

There are ethical issues involved in all types of writing. Medical writing has more than any other type.

Conflict of Interest

A conflict of interest occurs when a medical author has some tie to activities that could be perceived as influencing objectivity or veracity. Conflict of interest may be financial, as in receiving funding support for a project or accepting honoraria as a speaker for a pharmaceutical company. It may also include being a consultant, providing expert testimony, owning stock in a company, or actually being employed by a company that makes a product mentioned in an article. Conflicts may even involve family members, academic competition, and personal relationships. For example, on several occasions I have been requested to write reviews on books that I thought might be seen as competition to books that I edit; I returned these books to the journal editor with a note explaining my perceived conflict of interest. Because I write on medical topics I do not serve on the speaker panel for any pharmaceutical companies and I do not buy individual stocks of drug companies or surgical supply manufacturers.

Not only authors can have conflicts of interest. Peer reviewers and editors may also have ethical dilemmas; I discuss this in Chapter 10.

Project-Specific Industry Financial and Material Support

In discussions of conflict of interest, project-specific industry support for research is an important concern. The JAMA requires that all financial and material support for research and the work "be clearly and completely identified in the Acknowledgment. The role of the funding organization or sponsor in the design and conduct of the study, in the collection, analysis, and interpretation of the data, and in the preparation, review, or approval of the manuscript should be specified."[11]

Because this issue is so crucial, and at the risk of redundancy, I am next going to quote the ICMJE[4] on project specific industry support:

> Editors should require authors to describe the role of outside sources of project support, if any, in a study design; in the collection, analysis and interpretation of data; and in the writing of the report. If the supporting source had no such involvement, the authors should so state. Because the bias potentially introduced by the direct involvement of supporting agencies in research are analogous to methodological biases of other sorts (e.g., study design, statistical and psychological factors), the type and degree of the supporting agency should be described in the Methods section. Editors should also require disclosure of whether or not the supporting agency controlled or influenced the decision to submit the final manuscript for publication.

Plagiarism

I was in a writing workshop in which someone asked a medical book editor what he thought was the biggest problem he faced. His answer surprised me: plagiarism.

The clinician with a good article idea should write it up. Let's look at the sentence I just wrote. In the history of writing, I believe that it is mathematically possible that I am the first person to put those 11 words together in exactly this way. On balance, my 11-word sentence does not describe a brilliantly inventive thought, and a claim to being the first to write this sentence must remain a presumptive guess. However, and modesty aside, if you or any other author wishes to use my sentence you should make clear that it is a quotation from this book and give full credit to the source.

Recently there have been some headlines regarding authors in respected positions being accused of plagiarism. I have faith in the goodness of my fellow humans and I choose to believe that the errors made arose from doing research without noting carefully what were personal ideas and what were someone else's words. I think of this as "accidental plagiarism." Yes, such plagiarism is unacceptable, but you can see what happened. I suspect that accidental plagiarism is most likely to occur when authors depend on others (students or research assistants) to do their research for them.

The rules of using borrowed material and how to obtain permission are covered in Chapter 4. If the voice in your subconscious whispers that you may be using someone else's work inappropriately, listen carefully to the message.

Ghost and Honorary Authors

Flanagin et al[12] did a study of 809 corresponding authors (the author self-identified as the one to contact about an article) of articles published in JAMA, NEJM, and *Annals of Internal Medicine* plus three other peer-reviewed smaller-circulation journals that publish supplements (*American Journal of Cardiology, Americal Journal of Medicine,* and *American Journal of Obstetrics and Gynecology*). The authors found that 19% of articles had evidence of honorary authors,

11% had evidence of ghost authors, and 2% had evidence of both. Honorary authors were more prevalent in review articles than in research reports.

The journals in the study are among our best. The suspected prevalence of honorary and ghost authors is appalling, especially since authors published in these prestigious journals are generally respected academicians.

In commenting on the Flanagin et al study, I can only say: If you wrote it or otherwise contributed substantially, put your name on it. If not, do not allow yourself to be listed as an author.

PROBLEMS WITH STANCE

Both beginning and experienced medical authors can have problems with stance. By this I mean overstating or understating your conclusions, especially in research reports.

Overstatement and Hubris

Hubris is excessive self-confidence. It represents pride that may approach arrogance. It can take several forms. One manifestation of hubris is attempting to write far beyond your writing skills, professional experience, and available data. Editors can quickly sniff out when they are being shoveled a load of bad-smelling stuff. Another hubristic act is making confident statements about what the future holds, which you should not do in any medium that can be read a decade later.

The most common manifestation of overstatement and hubris occurs in presumptuous phrases, such as, "All physicians should ..." and "It should be apparent at this point that ..."

Table 5.4 lists more such words that should give you pause if you use them in your conclusions.

Understatement and Waffling

Just as bad as overstatement is understatement. By understating perfectly good work, you undermine your valid findings and your own credibility. Table 5.5 lists some words that

TABLE 5.4.   Hubristic words and phrases

Meaningful
Important
Key
Chief
Foremost
Consequential
Central
Essential
Substantial
Major finding
It is true that …
One must conclude that …
We can all agree that …

TABLE 5.5.   Waffle words and phrases

Possibly
Probably
Potentially
Perhaps
Maybe
Might
May
Apparently
It appears that …
It is conceivable that …
It is very possible that …

should alert you that you might be understating your conclusions.

WHAT MAKES A GREAT MEDICAL ARTICLE?

Chapters 6 through 10 discuss the various types of medical articles, chapters, and books. First, let's review what makes a great medical article:

■ *A topic of general interest.* Your topic must answer the questions, "So what?" and "Who cares?" The general medical reader is probably not interested in a rare tropical disease never seen in the U.S. or Europe, but may be interested if you can tell something new about problems in daily practice.

■ *Meaningful information about the topic.* I use the "Monday morning" question. If I read this article over the weekend, might it possibly be of help to me in the hospital or office Monday morning?

■ *Objectives clearly stated.* Tell your reader early in the article what to expect. This is especially important in a research report, in which the research question should be clearly articulated in the introduction.

■ *A structure that presents data clearly.* Don't start writing until you have the structural concept clearly in mind. The structure tells you and the reader where you are going. Of all aspects of the article, this is the most difficult to repair later.

■ *Articulate and authoritative prose.* Good data presented in bad prose may be rejected by a journal. King[13] has summarized the requirements for good expository writing in a single sentence: "Know what you want to say, say it clearly, and then stop." Be very selective in your use of long sentences, big words, and AAs.

■ *Tables and figures that complement the text.* Used judiciously, they can be the most important part of your article.

■ *A clear, concise title.* Label your work clearly and in a way that readers may recall later.

REFERENCES

1. Frey JJ. Elements of composition. In: Taylor RB, Munning KA, eds. Written communication in family medicine. New York: Springer-Verlag; 1984:4.
2. Wallechinsky D, Wallace I. The people's almanac. Garden City, NY: Doubleday; 1975:746.
3. Highet G. Explorations. New York: Oxford University Press; 1971:99.
4. International Committee of Medical Journal Editors. Uniform requirements for manuscripts submitted to biomedical journals. Available at: www.icmje.org.

5. Garfield E. Citation indexing. Its theory and applications in science, technology, and humanities. Philadelphia: ISI Press; 1979.

6. Impact factor of journals. Available at: http://www.nara-wu.ac.jp/life/food/mbio/impactfactor/2001_order.html.

7. Ojasoo T, Maisonneuve H, Matillon Y. The impact factor of medical journals, a biometric indicator to be handled with care (in French). Presse Med 2002;31(17):775–781.

8. Taylor RB. How physicians read the medical literature. Female Patient 2004;29(1):8–11.

9. Jordan EP, Shepard WC. Rx for medical writing. Philadelphia: WB Saunders; 1952:14.

10. Shem S. The house of God. New York: Dell; 1978.

11. Journal of the American Medical Association. Instructions for authors. Available at: http://jama.ama-assn.org/ifora_current/dtl.

12. Flanagin A, Carey LA, Fontanarosa PG, et al. Prevalence of articles with honorary authors and ghost writers in peer-reviewed medical journals. JAMA 1998;280:222–224.

13. King LS. Why not say it clearly? Boston: Little, Brown; 1978:109.

6

How to Write a Review Article

The review article is the Rodney Dangerfield of medical writing. Review articles get no respect. Yet, surprisingly, many respected academicians write review articles, for both subscriber-based and controlled-circulation journals. Why do they do so? The answer is that, by writing review articles, the academician clinicians assert their claims—mark their territory—on topics such as renin levels in hypertension or advances in the surgical management of hemorrhoids.

In addition to the fact that many are written by prestigious authors, another reason that review articles should get more respect is that they are usually very well written. When presenting a new way of organizing known data or discussing how to manage a certain problem in the office, the article must be skillfully composed if it is to hold the reader's attention. The reader must think that the content is worth reading. For this reason, most review articles are both peer reviewed for medical content and carefully edited to make them easy to read.

This will not be a long chapter because, by using the review article as an example of how to approach concept and structure, I have already covered several of the most important topics. In Chapter 2 I discussed general ways to develop an idea into the structure of an article, and in Chapter 3 I discussed how the idea and structural concept could be developed into an expanded outline. Chapter 4 covered how to construct tables, figures, and reference lists. Nevertheless, there are still some things to discuss about writing review articles.

ABOUT THE REVIEW ARTICLE

What Is the Review Article?

Fundamentally, the review paper is an essay. It has similarities to the essays you and I have been writing since junior high school: It has a topic, a beginning, development of the theme in a logical manner, and an ending. Some may hold that the review paper is not an original publication.[1] I understand the "nonoriginal" viewpoint, especially if held by a research scientist. It is true that review papers add no new data to the literature. However, I believe that review articles are original in that they bring new thinking to the literature. They provide us with practical insights and offer new approaches to old problems. In this way they are innovative and they expand medical understanding.

There are some various types of review articles. We are all familiar with the traditional review articles. Sometimes called clinical updates, traditional review articles bring together known facts in a meaningful way. Examples include how to approach a clinical problem such as "Subclinical Thyroid Disease: Clinical Applications" (JAMA 2004;291:239–243) and how to perform a procedure such as "Diaphragm Fitting" (Am Fam Physician 2004;69(1):97–100). In addition to the traditional types, there are specialized review articles that are discussed later in the chapter. These are the literature review discussing the state of the art, the meta-analysis, and the evidence-based clinical review.

Who Publishes Review Articles and Who Reads Them?

Who Publishes Review Articles?

Not all review articles are published in controlled-publication journals—the "throw-aways." Almost all journals, even the most prestigious ones, publish review articles regularly. They may carry a general label, such as "Review Article" as in the *New England Journal of Medicine* (NEJM), or "Review(s)" as in the *British Medical Journal for the American Physician* (BMJ-USA). Or they may be titled something more specific, such as "Clinician's Corner: Contempo Updates—Linking Evidence and Experience" in the *Journal of the American Medical Association* (JAMA).

The fact that virtually all journals publish review articles is favorable for the new author. If you write a thoughtful, well-organized article in competent prose, you should eventually see it in print. Realistically, your chances of success with the international "big four"—*The Lancet*, NEJM, JAMA, and BMJ—is not high, for the very good reason that these leading publications seek contributions from the world's leaders in each area.

Do not despair. The many refereed journals in your specialty and the dozens of broad-based controlled-circulation journals need a constant supply of review papers, and because of the ongoing need for good articles, they cannot wait until the world leader in the field decides to submit a review article. In the less prestigious journals, those with the lower impact factors (see Chapter 5), your chances of publication are good.

I recommend calling the journal editor first. An early discussion with the editor about your article idea can help avoid disappointment. It also establishes a personal relationship and helps assure an eventual favorable decision. Try for telephone contact whenever possible; an e-mail is a more impersonal second choice. Table 6.1 lists some journals that may be good targets for your article. The contact information may be different by the time you read this book: editors, telephone numbers, and e-mail addresses change. Try the listed contact information as a beginning, and then use "network research," as described in Chapter 3, to get the correct person on the line. If this fails, use Google to search for the journal name and then seek the editor's contact information. Later in the chapter, I will discuss how to structure your conversation with the editor.

Who Reads Review Articles?

The quick answer is, "Almost all clinicians." This includes not only physicians and scientists, but medical students, residents, and fellows. Other readers may be health policy experts and even attorneys. My review articles on headaches yield fairly frequent calls from attorneys across America, asking me to testify in professional liability cases involving patients with headaches.

As I noted in Chapter 5, readers often "graze" review articles. Some busy physicians save these articles to read as relaxation in the evening. Others take a pile of review article tear-outs to read on long plane rides or—not recommended—at the poolside on vacation.

TABLE 6.1. Selected journals that publish review articles

Advanced Studies in Medicine
  Johns Hopkins School of Medicine
  720 Rutland Avenue
  Baltimore, Maryland 21205
  Telephone: (908) 253-9001
  ljiorle@JHASIM.com
American Family Physician
  Publication Division
  American Academy of Family Physicians
  11400 Tomahawk Parkway
  Leawood, Kansas 66211-2672
  Telephone: (800) 274-223
  http://www.aafp.org
Consultant
  Cliggott Publishing
  330 Boston Post Road, Box 4027
  Darien, Connecticut 06820-4027
  Telephone: (203) 662-6400
  http://www.ConsultantLive.com
Cortlandt Forum
  114 West 26th Street, 3rd Floor
  New York, NY 10001
  Telephone: (646) 638-6117
  Editor@cortlandtforum.com
Emergency Medicine
  Quadrant HealthCom, Inc.
  26 Main Street
  Chatham, New Jersey 07928-2402
  Telephone: (973) 701-8900
  http://www.quadrantem@emscirc.com
Family Practice Recertification
  Medical World Business Press
  241 Forsgate Drive
  Jamesburg, New Jersey 08831-0505
  Telephone: (732) 656-1140
  http://e-mail: jmonaghan@mwc.com
The Female Patient
  Quadrant HealthCom, Inc.
  26 Main Street
  Chatham, New Jersey 07928-2402
  Telephone: (973) 701-2740
  e-mail: tracey.giannouris@qhc.com
Hospital Physician
  Turner White Communications, Inc.
  125 Strafford Ave., Suite 220
  Wayne, Pennsylvania 19087-3391
  Telephone: (610) 975-4541
  http://www.turner-white.com

(Contd)

TABLE 6.1. *(Contd)*

Infections in Medicine
    Cliggott Publishing
    330 Boston Post Road, Box 4027
    Darien, Connecticut 06820-4027
    Telephone: (203) 662-6582
    http://www.scp.com/content/JouPub/clgiimautguide.html

Journal of General Internal Medicine
    2501 M Street NW, Suite 575
    Washington, DC 20037
    Telephone: (800) 822-3060
    http://www.blackwellpublishing.com/journals

Postgraduate Medicine
    4530 West 77th Street
    Minneapolis, Minnesota 55435
    Telephone: (952) 835-3222
    http://www.pgmeditor@mcgraw-hill.com

Primary Psychiatry
    MBL Communications, Inc.
    333 Hudson Street, 7th Floor
    New York, New York 10013
    Telephone: (212) 328-0800
    http://www.primarypsychiatry.com

Reviews in Urology
    MedReviews, LLC
    1333 Broadway, Suite 400
    New York, New York 10018
    Telephone: (212) 971-4047
    http://www.medreviews.com

Western Journal of Medicine
    221 Main Street
    P.O. Box 7690
    San Francisco, California 94120-7690
    Telephone: (415) 974-5977
    e-mail:wjm@ewjm.com
    http://www.ewjm.com

Women's Health in Primary Care
    Jobson Publishing, LLC
    100 Avenue of the Americas
    New York, New York 10013-1678
    Telephone: (973) 916-1000
    http://www.jobson.com

Referral physicians also read review articles, and many nationally known specialists in narrow fields attribute some patient referrals to review articles that they have published in medical journals.

PLANNING A REVIEW ARTICLE

Getting Started

Let us begin with the premise that you would like to write a review article as a way of getting started in medical writing. What should you do next? First, I suggest that you review Chapters 2 and 3 about topic ideas and article development. Then, begin with the work you do each day, which may be seeing patients in the office, acting as a hospitalist for inpatients, performing surgery, or caring for elderly individuals in a nursing home. Within the scope of your work, find what intrigues you, and ask yourself, What have I learned in my years of practice that I would like to share with my colleagues?

Writing a review article soon becomes a learning exercise— for the author. There are two phases. First, you must learn whether anyone else has recently published the article you are planning to write. Do this by searching PubMed, MDConsult, Google, or your own favorite Web-searching site. Be cautious with your conclusion that you have happened upon virgin territory—a topic that no one has written about yet. There two reasons to suspect such a conclusion: There is a lag between publication and when you will find the report on the Web site, and some controlled-circulation journals are not indexed at all.

The second phase of learning comes as you learn more about your topic. This is the research phase, described earlier in Chapters 1 and 3. A fairly thorough search is useful early, even at the stage of deciding whether to write the article at all. It can avoid disappointment later.

Next comes thinking about how to handle your chosen topic.

How to Handle Your Topic

As you think about how to organize your article, it is often helpful to scan your target journal, and look at how authors

TABLE 6.2. Structure of selected review articles

Article title	Article concept and structure
Reproductive mood disorders (Prim Psych 2003;10(12):31–40)	Recognition and management of mood disorders in the perimenstrual time, in pregnancy and the postpartum period, and in the perimenopause
A review of common eyelid conditions for the primary care physician (Adv Stud Med 2003;3(10): 563–570)	Diagnosis and treatment of blepharoptosis (drooping upper eyelid) and four other conditions; several photos
Health effects of climate change (JAMA 2004;291:99–103)	An overview of the health effects of heat waves, floods and droughts, air pollution, water-related diseases, and more
Heart failure: update on therapeutic options (Consultant 2003;43(14): 1649–1654)	An overview of what experts now consider optimum therapy with beta-blockers, ACE inhibitors, diuretics, angiotensin receptor blockers, and more
Update on vaccinations for women (The Female Patient 2004;29(1): 12–18)	A discussion of inoculations women need at various stages of life
How to assess and treat erectile dysfunction (Emerg Med 2004;36(1): 28–37)	Uses traditional review article headings of "pathophysiology," "causes," "diagnosis," and "therapy"

there have organized what they wanted to say. Let us now look at some published review articles to see how the authors dealt with their material (Table 6.2).

I did not need to search very far to find the examples in Table 6.2. Publications containing traditional review articles such as the ones listed cross our desks every day. Let's look at the ways the listed examples approached their subjects: The reproductive mood disorders article used life changes to cluster mood disorders. Five selected conditions are discussed in the eyelid disorders article. In the article on heat effects of climate change, the authors grouped problems under various types of environmental problem. The heart failure review article lists and discusses the medications used. The vaccinations for women article discusses immunizations for nonpregnant and pregnant women, using one table and two charts. The erectile dysfunction article in *Emergency Medicine* presents a textbook overview of the problem, but leaves unanswered why this is an emergency problem.

In each instance, the authors were writing on areas in which they worked each day. They believed that they had something useful to share with colleagues, and they organized their articles in ways that may help us remember the points made.

Consulting with the Journal Editor

As I mentioned briefly above, I urge that you contact the journal editor, preferably by telephone. This call can help you better understand the editorial process. Making personal contact with a journal editor can not only help with the current article; it can be the beginning of a relationship that can be useful in the future. Medical journalism is a relatively small community, and medical editors often change jobs from one publisher to another. Several of my good friends today are medical editors with whom I have worked on various projects as they have moved from one publishing job to another.

Contacting the editor can also save you hours of wasted effort. It is not a good idea to prepare a review article for a favorite journal and submit the manuscript, only to have the editor reply that they have a very similar article scheduled for publication next month.

When you call the editor you should be prepared to discuss the following:

- The topic and how you will handle the subject matter
- Why you are qualified to write on this topic
- How many tables or figures you plan for the article
- When the manuscript will be completed
- If you have any possible conflict of interest.

Most editors are able to give you an encouraging or discouraging answer over the telephone, which is all they can do at this time. The editor usually cannot promise acceptance without seeing the completed article. As an interim step, the editor may request to see an outline showing major headings.

If you submit an outline, I suggest adding a copy of your abbreviated curriculum vitae.

SPECIAL TYPES OF REVIEW ARTICLE

There are three special types of review article. The literature review is usually recognizable, but not always. The boundaries between the evidence-based clinical review and the meta-analysis are often not clear.

Literature Review

The literature review is written to discuss the state of the art. Sometimes the authors use the words *literature, review,* or *state of the art* in the title. If not, you can usually recognize a literature review by the general title, and the absence of the words such as *study of, surveillance of,* or *effects of.* Another tip-off that you are looking at a literature review is a long list of references, in the general range of 100, perhaps more.

In the world of medical writing, literature reviews serve several useful purposes:

- To summarize research on a topic as a bridge to applied use. That is, to present data for those who are not actively involved in the field, but who need to know the latest information to provide good patient care.
- To synthesize knowledge as a springboard for future research.
- To support academic rigor in a field.
- To serve as a database for health policy decisions.

An example of literature reviews is a recent article titled "Diabetic Retinopathy," presenting a discussion of clinical and histopathological manifestations, prevention and treatment, experimental therapies, genetic influences, and new diagnostic methods in regard to diabetic retinopathy. The article has 95 reference citations (N Engl J Med 2004;350:48–59).

In 2004, JAMA published a state-of-the-art review titled, "Neuroprotection in Parkinson Disease: Mysteries, Myths, and Misconceptions," with a restrained reference list of only

58 citations (JAMA 2004;291:358–364). This article, with its alliterative title, is probably a literature review, but some may argue that it is a traditional review article.

In the *Journal of General Internal Medicine* (JGIM) is an article titled, "Detection, Evaluation, and Treatment of Eating Disorders: The Role of the Primary Care Physician." What brought this article to my attention was the structured abstract with the headings: Objective, Design, Measurements and Main Results, and Conclusion. So far the abstract could be summarizing a research article. The tip-off that this is a review article is that, in the body of the abstract, the design is described as "A review of the literature from … ," and the conclusion is a single sentence: "Primary care providers have an important role in detecting and managing eating disorders" (JGIM 2000; 15(8):577–582).

Another example of the state-of-the-art literature review is a thoughtful article titled "Defining and Measuring Interpersonal Continuity of Care" (Ann Fam Med 2003;1:134–143). This is a literature review of 146 reports on the topic of continuity of care in the clinical setting. The authors provide analysis based on the commonality of findings in various diverse articles. And so the question arises: Is this article best described as a literature review or a meta-analysis?

The literature review is not very difficult to write. Modern computer technology makes assembling 100 papers on a topic merely a morning's work. In this and earlier chapters I have told you how to develop a concept and convert it into an outline. There is no reason why the beginning writer cannot create a credible state-of-the-art literature review.

There is, however, another difficulty that must be faced. A leading expert in the field usually writes the state-of-the-art literature review on a clinical topic. Add to this fact the reality that literature reviews are usually long articles—by this I mean more than 20 double-spaced manuscript pages. It takes a lot of space to describe the state of the art on any topic. And so, when presented with a long article by an unknown author, the journal editor will look carefully to see if you are qualified to present the state of the art to the journal's readers.

I do not wish to discourage you from writing literature reviews, but I suggest that such an effort should be done under the tutelage of a nationally know mentor, or perhaps postponed until you are a recognized author on your career topic.

Meta-Analysis

Meta-analysis is a method of combining the results of several studies into a summary conclusion, using quantitative strategies that will allow consideration of data in diverse research reports. It is a special type of systematic review intended to answer a focused clinical question.[2] In a sense, meta-analysis is a research study about research studies. Writing a meta-analysis review paper calls for a knowledge of statistical methods that is beyond the scope of this book, and that is beyond the skill set of most clinician authors. This means that, if you are as statistically challenged as most of us, you should not undertake a meta-analysis without a close collaborative relationship with a coauthor who is well trained in statistical analysis.

As mentioned above, the boundaries between state-of-the-art reviews and the meta-analysis can sometimes be murky. Most easily recognizable are the meta-analyses that are so identified by the authors in the title. For example, consider the helpful title, "Arterial Puncture Closing Devices Compared with Standard Manual Compression After Cardiac Catheterization: Systematic Review and Meta-Analysis" (JAMA 2004;291; 350–357). The four authors are very clear on what you will find in the article. In JGIM is another example of a clearly titled article: "Meta-Analysis of Vascular and Neoplastic Events Associated with Tamoxifen" (J Gen Intern Med 2003;18:937–947). The JGIM article reports on 32 trials (52,929 patients) with one or more outcomes of interest.

The abstracts of both of the examples cited above cite relative risk, confidence intervals, and data that are very reminiscent of reports of original research. The JAMA instructions for authors[3] state, "Manuscripts reporting results of meta-analyses should include an abstract of no more than 300 words using the following headings: Context, Objective, Data Sources, Study Selection, Data Extraction, Data Synthesis, and Conclusions." Explanations of what to include in each category are on the Web site.

Some are likely to argue that the meta-analysis is research and should not be considered a review article at all. The tendency to consider meta-analysis as a type of research places special burdens on authors. By this I mean that conclusions must be supported clearly by data, and not by opinion. An article in the *Archives of Surgery* set out to explore this hypothesis: "A review of the literature will show that laparoscopy is safe and effective for the treatment of surgical diseases in elderly patients" (Arch Surg 2003;138:1083–1088). The authors selected "all relevant studies that could be obtained..." Their search covered three procedures: laparoscopic cholecystectomy (16 studies), laparoscopic antireflux surgery (four studies), and laparoscopic colon resection (10 reports). Okay so far. Their conclusions, however, seem to me to move beyond the data: "Despite underlying co-morbidities, individuals older than 65 years tolerate laparoscopic procedures extremely well. Complications and hospitalization are lower than in open procedures. Surgeons need to inform primary care physicians of the excellent result of laparoscopic procedures in the elderly to encourage early referrals." Can we generalize from three procedures to all laparoscopic procedures in the elderly? Maybe yes, maybe no. The articles studied addressed surgical outcomes such as symptom relief and cardiopulmonary morbidity. Did the 30 studies have anything to do with informing primary physicians? Also, although there were generally better surgical outcomes when laparoscopic procedures were compared with open surgery, did the 30 studies show that early referrals are beneficial to the patient? A meta-analysis about safety and efficacy of a procedure seems to have evolved to conclusions that might strike some readers as marketing.

Evidence-Based Clinical Review

The evidence-based clinical review is a special type of meta-analysis that is focused on a clinically relevant question. The emphasis is on evidence-based medicine (EBM) studies, which can be found through sites such as those listed in Table 6.3.

Evidence-based clinical reviews pay special attention to the quality of the studies included for analysis. The U.S.

TABLE 6.3. Evidence-based medicine (EBM) sources on the Web

Resource	Web site
Agency for Healthcare Research and Quality (AHRQ), previously known as the Agency for Health Care Policy and Research (AHCPR): a good source for clinical guidelines and evidence reports	http://www.ahrq.gov/clinic
Bandolier: contains summaries of articles on EBM	http://www.jr2.ox.ac.uk/bandolier
Clinical Evidence, BMJ Publishing Group: presents general EBM information, EBM tools, and summaries of evidence: registration is required	http://www.clinicalevidence.org
Cochrane Database of Systematic Review: contains systematic reviews from the Cochrane Collaboration	http://www.cochrane.org
Effective Health Care Bulletins: bimonthly peer-reviewed publication on EBM	http://www.york.ac.uk/inst/cdr/ehcb.htm
Institute for Clinical Systems Improvement (ICSI): good site for disease management and prevention guidelines	http://www.ICSI.org
Netting the Evidence: offers access to EBM organizations and learning resources, such as EBM software and virutal library	http://www.nettingtheevidence.org.uk
Primary Care Clinical Practice Guidelines, courtesy of University of California, San Francisco: includes links to articles, organizations, and EBM sites	http://www.medicine@ucsf.edu/resources
United States Preventive Services Task Force: presents up-to-date preventive services clinical recommendations, based on systematic reviews	http://www.ahrq.gov/clinic/uspstfix.htm

Preventive Services Task Force has been a leader in pointing out that study quality matters, and that the internal validity of a study is an important consideration as well as looking at whether the authors reported a randomized clinical trial, cohort, or case–control study.[4]

The journal *American Family Physician* has been a leader in advocating for the evidence-based clinical review article. This journal asks authors of evidence-based clinical review articles to "rate the level of evidence for key recommendations according to the following scale: level A [randomized controlled trial (RCT), meta-analysis]; level B (other evidence); level C (consensus/expert opinion). Siwek et al[2] have written an excellent paper that I recommend to anyone planning to write an evidence-based clinical review article. A more recent paper presents a strength of recommendation taxonomy (SORT) to grade evidence in the medical literature.[5]

MISTAKES WE MAKE WHEN WRITING REVIEW ARTICLES

We go wrong writing review article in predictable ways. Since the review article is the first project many beginning medical writers undertake, I think it is useful to summarize some of the mistakes we make as beginners. In thinking about it, some of us more experienced authors continue to make some of these errors:

- *Unimportant topic*: Do not waste effort writing a review article on a topic that no one cares about. Field-test your idea with colleagues in the office or hospital. If you are planning to write a *How to do it* article on a new way to recognize borderline personality disorder or a procedure to trim hypertrophic toenails, ask several colleagues whether they might be interested in reading such an article.
- *Stale rehash*: Be sure that you are saying something new about the topic. Step one is a literature search. Step two is a call to a journal editor. Take these steps to avoid writing an article that is not publishable.
- *A timely topic, but already covered*: The call to the editor of your journal may reveal that your timely topic, such as a sharply rising trend in elective cesarean sections, is such a great idea that an article is already in press. You may change your target journal. Certainly you have gained useful information.
- *Getting lost along the way*: Make an outline with major headings, and stick to it.

■ *Article too long*: Some editors say that this is one of the most common problems in medical writing. Why is it, with writing being such hard work, that we all tend to over-write? Review articles should generally be about 16 to 20 double-spaced manuscript pages, total including references. State-of-the-art literature reviews are the exception, and may be longer.

■ *Too many or too few references*: Avoid this mistake by studying similar articles published in your target journal.

SUMMARY

This chapter has been much like a review article; it had an introduction, topic development using four major headings, a summary, and a few references. In fact, this chapter could, with very little modification, be published as a journal article. The point is that classic review articles and book chapters are much alike.

There are also similarities among review articles and case reports, editorials, letters, and book reviews. On the other hand, there are important differences among these article types. In the next chapter, I discuss four more writing models.

REFERENCES

1. Day RA. How to publish a scientific paper. 5th ed. Westport, CT: Oryx; 1998:163.
2. Siwek J, Gourlay ML, Slawson DC, Shaughnessy AF. How to write an evidence-based clinical review article. Am Fam Phys 2002;65:251–258.
3. Journal of the American Medical Association. Instructions for authors. JAMA 2004;291:125–131. Available at: http://jama.ama-assn.org/ifora_current/dtl.
4. Harris RP, Helfand M, Wolff SH, et al. Methods Work Group, Third U.S. Preventive Services Task Force. Current methods of the U.S. Preventive Services Task Force. A review of the process. Am J Prev Med 2001;20(3 suppl):21–35.
5. Ebell MH, Siwek J, Weiss BD, et al. Strength of recommendation taxonomy (SORT): a patient-centered approach to grading evidence in the medical literature. Am Fam Phys 2004; 69:548–556.

7

Case Reports, Editorials, Letters to the Editor, Book Reviews, and Other Publication Models

Several writing models yield products with fewer pages than the typical review article. This does not mean that they are any easier to write or to get published. Most submissions will be peer reviewed, and there is the inevitable competition for space in every journal. However, for many clinicians, the case report, book review, or practice tip may turn out to be the pathway to an early publication on their curriculum vitae. Each of the models described has different characteristics and requirements.

CASE REPORT

As stated by Jordan and Shepard,[1] "The case report occupies a peculiar and deserved role among medical articles. Many worthwhile clinical observations do not lend themselves to controlled or scientific study but deserve recording and contribute to medical advance." For most of us the urge to report a case occurs when we encounter a disease manifestation or therapeutic outcome that lies so far outside our familiar realm of experience that we feel compelled to share the observation with others.

One cannot set out today to write a case report without a case. I might decide this weekend to write a review article about unusual types of primary headaches or an editorial about why we clinicians should receive more pay for what we do. But to write a case report I need a patient with a disease, and then I must sense that there is something unusual about what I have observed.

When considering writing a case report, your next task is a literature review. In many cases you will find that what you have found is not nearly as uncommon as you originally believed. Just because you have first encountered an unexpected side effect of a drug, for example, does not mean that this side effect has not been seen and reported by many others. Prior reporting of your observation, in itself, need not prevent you from writing the report. What makes a great case report is the case-related analysis that advances our collective medical knowledge.

In a sense, the case report is a focused review article. What is different is the emphasis on one or more actual cases, with a rationale for why the findings are being reported, and an evidence-based analysis of what has been found. For example, Mainville and Connolly report an instance of acute visual loss after initiation of antihypertensive therapy with fosinopril and hydrochlorothiazide. The authors really don't know why the 50-year-old patient experienced the unilateral visual loss, but the event served as a springboard to an excellent discussion of central retinal artery occlusion, giant cell arteritis, and other causes of sudden visual loss (Mainville N, Connolly WES. Acute visual loss after initiation of antihypertensive therapy: case report. Can Med Assoc J 2003;169(4):313–315).

I think that highest accolades go to those case reports that change what we do in practice. For example, in 2001 Muench and Carey reported a case of a 38-year-old patient with schizophrenia who suddenly developed diabetes mellitus and ketoacidosis 12 months after starting the atypical antipsychotic medication olanzapine. The authors note that, including their case, there have been 30 such reports in the literature. What is noteworthy, in my opinion, is that on November 10, 2003, my clinician colleagues and I received a "Dear Healthcare Provider" letter from a pharmaceutical manufacturer stating that, "The Food and Drug Administration (FDA) has requested all manufacturers of atypical antipsychotics to include a warning regarding hyperglycemia and diabetes mellitus in their product labeling." (Muench J, Carey M. Diabetes mellitus associated with atypical antipsychotic medications: new case report and review of the literature. J Am Board Fam Pract 2001;14:278–282; and Letter from Janssen Pharmaceutica, Inc., dated November 10, 2003). This report and others on this topic appear to have prompted FDA action.

Types of Case Report

There are fundamentally two types of case report. The first is the observation of some unusual disease manifestation occurring in a single patient. For most clinicians, this is your most likely pathway to a case report. One example is a report of an unusual lesion of the finger in a 53-year-old man, with some excellent color photos (Meyerle JH, Keller RA, Krivda SJ. Superficial acral fibromyxoma of the index finger. J Am Acad Dermatol 2004;50(1):134–135). Diagnostic images or photographs greatly enhance the "single-patient" case report. In the end, this type of report must derive its value from the novelty of the finding, and the perception that other physicians should be aware of your case.

The second type of case report includes more than one observation. It may be several patients with an uncommon disease, such as an increased incidence of leukemia in a single neighborhood. Or perhaps you have recently encountered three young adult patients with hypnic headache. Your case report will describe the characteristics of what may be an evolving disease cluster or a new manifestation of a known disease.

Format for the Case Report

Itskowitz and Lebovitz report a case of a 77-year-old woman who was not taking antibiotics and who nevertheless developed pseudomembranous colitis (PMC) (Itskowitz MS, Lebovitz PJ. Nonantibiotic-associated pseudomembranous colitis: a case report and review of the literature. Adv Stud Med 2003;3(10):571–574). In their article the authors present the classic format for a case report:

- *Introduction*: The first paragraph discusses why the case is unusual: "Almost all cases of PMC reported during the past 3 decades have been associated with antimicrobial use." In my opinion, this is a valid justification for the report. As a practicing clinician, I need to know that nonantibiotic-associated PMC can occur.
- *Case description*: The authors present the relevant data, including medical history, physical findings, results of tests and procedures, and treatment received.

- *Literature review*: Nine instances of nonantibiotic PMC were found in the literature.
- *Discussion*: Here the authors discuss microflora of the intestine and other possible causes of PMC.
- *Conclusion*: What it all means is this: "When more common causes of acute enteritis and colitis have been ruled out, PMC should be considered in patients who develop persistent diarrhea, even without a history of antibiotic use."
- *References*: Sixteen references are listed. I think this number is about right. The case report is not intended to be a state-of-the-art literature review.

The case report should not be too long. If your case report exceeds 12 double-spaced manuscript pages, consider cutting.

Never claim to have elucidated a new syndrome. Such hubris will be severely criticized. If you have, in fact, found the first case ever of jejunal pregnancy, your colleagues—not you—should record your primacy.

EDITORIAL

Editorials are fun to write. They are generally short, and thus do not take weeks of labor. They rely on your experience and intuition, and thereby don't call for a major research effort. And they allow you to express your opinion. Unfortunately, not too many beginning writers have the chance to write and publish editorials. But some are successful.

The term *editorial* comes from *editor*, in turn derived from the French word *editeur*, actually meaning publisher.[2] The connotation is that the writing is by the publisher, the editor, or a designated authority. The topic usually reflects the individual's opinion, and today you may see the term *op-ed*, short for opinion-editorial. Today, editors are busy producing budgets and correcting errors of careless authors, and they often lack the specialized knowledge to produce the expert content needed, so they do not write all editorials.

There are fundamentally two types of editorial: those invited by the editor or publisher and those that are volunteered. Invited editorials may be focused, as in an invitation to comment on a specific research study being published, or the invitation may be open-ended: "Would you care to write an editorial for a coming issue of the journal?" These open-ended invitations usually are extended to prestigious members of the journal's editorial board.

Most journals publish editorials; the October 2001 issue of *British Medical Journal* (BMJ)-USA had five—count 'em, five—editorials. Your best chance of having an editorial published is to submit a brilliantly written opinion piece on a topic about which you have special knowledge. For example, those of us who practice in Oregon have enjoyed a unique opportunity with the Oregon Health Plan. This innovative plan explicitly rations health care to needy patients according to "the list," a catalog of diagnosis–treatment pairs laboriously negotiated with attention to fairness and to efficacy of interventions. A number of Oregon physicians have written editorials about this plan, with their chief authority being that they are practicing Oregon clinicians.

Your best chance of having an editorial published is to be asked to write a clinical commentary, which is generally a short opinion piece that accompanies a research article. It discusses how the research findings relate to actual practice (see below).

Some Types of Editorial

Editorial Salesmanship

Such editorials are really prefaces to an issue of the journal. They usually begin, "In this issue of the journal, we present ..." Then the editor goes on to discuss why they chose to publish the five studies on amino acids in rat livers that occupy the pages that follow.

The Editor's Opinion

In the January 31, 2004, issue of the BMJ, editor Richard Smith contrasted his journal with the *Economist*, in the sense that we clinicians "merely" deal with health issues, while at a World Economic Forum held in the Swiss ski resort of Davos each year, political leaders and economists can claim to be "committed to improving the state of the world." He concludes,

"Health must now—and perhaps for ever—take a subservient place to lofty goals" (Smith R. Economics first; health third, fourth, or nowhere. BMJ 2004;328:0). Here Dr. Smith discusses his opinion about where medicine stands in the paradigm he describes. As editor, he has the prerogative to state his opinion; readers are free to agree or disagree. In fact, I suspect that Dr. Smith will be most happy if his editorial provokes vigorous discussion.

Editorial Comment Regarding a Published Study

"I feel honored to have been asked to comment on this excellent article, 'Palliative Care in the Surgical Intensive Unit.'" This is the first sentence in an "invited commentary" editorial. The author of the commentary goes on to link a current case report to some published articles and his own personal experience (Civetta JM. Invited commentary. J Am Coll Surg 2002;194(1):83–85).

A *New England Journal of Medicine* (NEJM) article on computed tomographic virtual colonoscopy (Pickhardt PJ, et al. Computed tomographic virtual colonoscopy to screen for colorectal neoplasia. NEJM 2003;349:2191–2200) is accompanied by an editorial on the state of the art of screening virtual colonoscopy (Morrin MM, LaMont JT. Screening virtual colonoscopy. NEJM 2003;349:2261–2263).

As mentioned above, this type of editorial offers opportunity for the clinician to offer a "front-line" viewpoint. I suggest that practicing clinicians write to the editors of their favorite journals, offering to write "invited commentary" related to research articles accepted for publication. Be sure that your letter is very well written, since this and the curriculum vitae that you include are the evidence the editor considers in deciding whether or not to invite you to contribute.

Sharing Special Insight

In the *Journal of General Internal Medicine* (JGIM), Singer writes about homelessness as a health hazard (Singer J. Taking it to the streets: homelessness, health, and health care in the United States. JGIM 2003;18:964–965). The author, unknown to me, lists his name and address as Jeff Singer, MSW, Health Care for the Homeless, Inc., Baltimore, MD. I strongly suspect that Mr. Singer has firsthand knowledge of the problems described in his editorial.

Sometimes a journal editor requests an editorial from an individual known to have a special viewpoint on a controversial topic. The journal can then publish the editorial, with the disclaimer that the opinion expressed is that of the author and does not necessarily reflect the opinion of the journal or publisher. Nevertheless, the journal editor got what was wanted in print.

Writing an Editorial

Classically, an editorial is a critical argument.[3] As such it should develop the thesis in a logical manner:

- *Present the problem.* Early in the first paragraph, tell your reader the issue you are addressing. The first sentence is a good place to do this. An exception may be the use of a vignette to introduce the problem, sometimes called "the hook" in nonmedical writing. For example, the editorial on homelessness as a health hazard (mentioned above) begins, "Jim, a Korean War veteran in his seventies, lives in a '79 Cadillac. Unable to afford housing, his hygiene is quite poor; access to water is limited to restaurant bathrooms ... "
- *Offer evidence to support your opinion.* Here is where you should visit the literature and offer an evidence-based argument. Select your references carefully, to avoid allowing your editorial to become a review article.
- *Offer personal insight.* What you are writing is, after all, your own opinion. It is okay to say what you think. It is even better to back up this opinion with a personal anecdote.
- *Offer counterevidence.* Not everyone will agree with you. Present the other side of the issue in an unbiased and respectful manner, and then say why you are not convinced.
- *Provide a summary.* A single closing paragraph is usually all that is needed at this point. Describe your conclusion, ideally relating what you write here to what you said in paragraph one. Perhaps include the implications of your conclusion to practice or to society. Then stop.

■ *Cite references*. I rarely write an editorial without references, but I only include a few.

■ *Include headings*. Your editorial may include headings to break up the flow of prose and to help the reader remember the structure of your article. Headings are especially useful for long editorials.

LETTER TO THE EDITOR

In January 1904, more than 100 years ago, a reader identified only as E.G. wrote to the JAMA editor, "Your editorial Jan. 9, 1904, discussing why scientists are poor writers, aroused my spirit of refutation, because I think your point is not well taken..." (E.G. Why are scientists poor writers? (letter). JAMA 1904;42:470,477). Today, letters to the editor are very popular, with both readers and publishers.

Most journals publish letters to the editor, and journal editors are pleased when there is lively discussion in the "Letters" column, as readers indulge their spirit of refutation and debate the merits of published articles. Sometimes they share new ideas. Some journals such as the BMJ are beginning to post letters online, allowing a "Rapid Response" by readers. The *Journal of the American Board of Family Practice* invites comments about JABFP articles as "Rapid Responses," which are posted on the Web site within days of submission.

Letters to the editor are a wonderful vehicle for the aspiring medical writer. There is no requirement that the author be a distinguished professor, no original research study is needed, and there is a reasonable chance of publication, at least in the journals that have limited readership. LaVigne[4] advocates this type of writing model: "Letters to the editor merit your consideration as a publication option: first, because letters and short pieces stand a better chance of being published than longer articles, and second, because published letters to the editor generally are titled and indexed, thus making them retrievable as articles in the journal."

The academic clinician will note that, even though letters are not refereed, published letters are indexed and are thus legitimate entries on a curriculum vitae. Whether or not one should list "rapid responses" on one's curriculum vitae is problematic.

Types of Letter

There are many types of letter to the editor. Here are some of them:

Attaboy

A member of the Academic Unit of Anaesthesia and Intensive Care of the University of Aberdeen, Scotland, wrote commenting on a paper published in *Critical Care Medicine*. The letter begins, "I would like to congratulate Dr. Dellinger for an excellent overview of cardiovascular management of septic shock." The letter concludes, "This is a very useful clinical review in the management of a condition with a high mortality rate, and I would certainly use this decision tree in my clinical practice" (Pravinkumar E. Letter: cardiovascular management of septic shock. Crit Care Med 2004;32(1):315).

In my opinion, such a letter written by the average clinician has little chance of being published. In fact, I really don't think that the author added anything to our fund of medical knowledge, and probably the journal space could have been better used in some other way.

New Idea to Add

As a practicing clinician you may have a thought that expands the knowledge presented in an article. Perhaps you have seen an illustrative case, and your fellow clinicians would benefit from the knowledge. In response to an article in *American Family Physician* (AFP) about management of diabetic foot ulcers, two readers wrote to add the following: "An effective adjunctive therapy for wound debridement that was not mentioned is maggot therapy" (Summers JB, Kaminski J. Letter: maggot debridement therapy for diabetic necrotic foot. AFP 2003;68(12):2327). They support their addition with a clear discussion and six references.

Disagreement

Sometimes readers just must disagree with something written in an article. Two readers contributed a letter to the

American Journal of Obstetrics and Gynecology, discussing the conclusions of a published research study on body mass index (BMI) and first trimester pregnancy outcomes in infertile patients. The readers write: "The authors finally concluded that outcome of singleton pregnancies in patients with infertility was not influenced by BMI. We disagree with these results" (Bellver J, Pellicer A. Letter: impact of obesity on spontaneous abortion. Am J Obstet Gynecol 2004;190:293).

Statement of Concern
The *Annals of Emergency Medicine* published an epidemiologic (case–control) study of homicide and suicide risks associated with firearms in the home. A reader writes to question the author's affiliations: "I doubt the *Annals'* editorial board would have published without commentary an article by a pro-gun organization purporting to defend gun ownership. The author's affiliations with anti-gun 'research' groups are no less compelling an argument for bias" (Fritz DA. Letter: lies, damned lies, and statistics. Ann Emerg Med 2004;43(1):141). This letter was accompanied, on the same page of the journal, by a reply written by the allegedly "anti-gun" article author.

Sounding Off
This type of letter is really a short editorial. Without reference to any published article, a reader wrote to discuss the issue of standard of care. "Medicine is not exact, and bad outcomes happen. The notion that physicians can follow a formula and avoid successful litigation is false" (Grant DC. Letter: I don't want to hear about the "standard of care." Ann Emerg Med 2004;43(1):139).

Uninvited "Sounding Off" letters must be timely, pertinent, and very well written if they are to be published. This statement is especially true if your name is not well known in medicine.

Gotcha
In response to an article about the use of low-dose colchicine in gout, a pharmacist writes that the authors "discussed the use of low dose colchicine in gout. The treatment dose of colchicine, which has remained at 1 mg initially, followed by 500 mcg every 2–3 hours for many years, should be reviewed.

However, they are incorrect to say that the current BNF (British National Formulary) recommends a regimen for colchicine that is unchanged since the 1966 edition. In September 1999 the BNF reduced the total dose of a course of colchicine from 10 to 6 mg. Before 1981 the BNF did not even state the higher limit of 10 mg" (Cox AR. Letter: colchicine in acute gout. BMJ 2004;328:288). Gotcha!

Transformed Research or Case Report

Whenever I read a case report or an account of original research presented as a letter to the editor, I often pause to reflect that the letter probably began life as a full article. As a full article, it was submitted and peer reviewed. The authors endured a few rejections by prestigious journals, until a sympathetic editor suggested that, if the findings could be shortened to 500 to 600 words, the work could be published as a letter. In football, this is the equivalent of an 85-yard drive with multiple first downs, and then settling for a field goal. With understandable ambivalence, the authors cut the article mercilessly, and accepted publication of their case or research report as a letter to the editor.

Writing the Letter

The successful letter to the editor is often more inspiration than perspiration. The urge to write a letter will often strike you when reading a journal article, and you think: I know something about this topic or have an opinion I want to share. You then do some research and the letter, which should be fairly short, will seem to write itself. Of course, as mentioned above, some letters do not comment on published articles.

Think of the letter to the editor as a very short combination of an editorial and a literature review. Limit yourself to making a single point. Do not try to combine two or more ideas into a short letter. In writing, you should select each word with care to stay within tight limits imposed by most journals. Even though you are likely to be acting upon an inspirational urge, you must craft your letter with great care if it is to be accepted for publication.

Most letters to the editor comment on published articles. In these instances, there is a general structure that the letter should follow:

- *Identify the paper.* In the first sentence, cite the paper that is the subject of your comments. This becomes your Reference 1.
- *State why you are writing.* State your agreement, disagreement, concern, or other reason for writing.
- *Give evidence.* The evidence may be from the literature or from personal experience. Literature-based evidence is better.
- *Provide a summary statement.* Conclude by tying all the above together.
- *Cite references.* Often a letter to the editor will have a few reference citations, but not too many.

Do not begin writing without reading the instructions to authors for the journal. Most instructions list requirements for submitted letters. The *Journal of the American Medical Association* (JAMA), for example, states, "Letters discussing a recent JAMA article should be received within 4 weeks of the article's publication and should not exceed 400 words of text and 5 references. Research letters reporting original research, including case series or case reports, also are welcome and should not exceed 600 words of text and 6 references, and may include a table or figure."[5]

JAMA prefers that letters be submitted electronically, and the *Annals of Emergency Medicine* no longer accepts letter submissions by mail.

The letter to the editor should be submitted just as you would a review paper. That means that you should begin with a title, and then prepare the manuscript double spaced on plain background, i.e., not on a letterhead. The letter manuscript should then be sent with a cover letter indicating that you are submitting the letter for publication and not merely to communicate with the editor. You should mention any special attributes that qualify you to write on the topic and reveal any potential conflicts of interest.

One final caution: If you are personally acquainted with the author of the article you plan to discuss in your letter, you may not want to write at all. If you praise the study, your friendship may impair your credibility. Worse, if you criticize the study, your comments may be interpreted as a personal attack.

BOOK REVIEW

Many, but not all, journals publish book reviews. Such reviews are a regular feature in NEJM and BMJ. JAMA expands the concept to review "Books, Journals, New Media." Some specialty and controlled-circulation journals carry book reviews in each edition; others do so intermittently. Not all reviews are of medical reference and textbooks: In January 2004, JAMA published a review of a television miniseries titled "Mavericks, Miracles, and Medicine" broadcast in four 1-hour segments on the History Channel. Reviews of medical software are now commonly seen.

The NEJM has published a review of *Breathing for a Living*, a memoir of a young woman who died at age 22 of cystic fibrosis. In the same December 2003 issue of NEJM is a review of *The Healing Art: A Doctor's Black Bag of Poetry. Prescription for Greed*, a novel by a well-known retired medical school professor and his son, a behavioral psychologist, was reviewed in JAMA in May 2001. So the books reviewed are not all scientific.

The journal editor or the journal's book review editor almost always invites book reviews. Occasionally an eager writer submits an unsolicited book review, but I doubt that many are published. Unsolicited reviews are suspect and editors need not take chances.

On the other hand, it is not too difficult to become a book reviewer. Any literate clinician can volunteer. Do so by identifying your one or two chief areas of clinical expertise, and then write to the journal editor offering your services. If selected to write a review, you will receive a copy of the book, which is yours to keep as payment for your contribution.

Book reviews are appropriate entries on your academic curriculum vitae.

Types of Book Review

Technically speaking, there are not different types of book review, but there are different approaches to the task. They are not mutually exclusive and more than one can be used in a single review. Whatever your approach(es), construct your book review with the same care and economy of words that you would devote to a review paper or research report.

Review in Relationship to the Author's Stated Purpose

I believe that all reviews should include this approach. I am a book author and editor, and I always begin my preface with a description of the intent of the book. I do so for the reviewer, as well as the reader. I earnestly hope that the reviewer will judge my work against my intention, and not against the book the reviewer wishes I had written. Also, as a reviewer, do not review the book in comparison with the book that you wish *you* had written.

Stedman's Medical Dictionary, 27th edition, for example, intends to provide "a comprehensive, current and accurate medical lexicon to medical and health professionals." This is a clearly stated goal, and if writing a review, I might ask: Is the book comprehensive? Is it current? Is it accurate? Is it written in a style appropriate for its audience of medical and health professionals?

A review of a book on cross-cultural medicine is summarized as follows: "Because Cross-Cultural Medicine is presented from the perspective of internal medicine, its many examples may not resonate as well with other physicians. However, *it meets its stated purpose* of providing 'internists with a framework for practicing culturally competent care' in a clear and succinct fashion" (italics added) (Moy E. Review of Bigby J. Cross-cultural medicine [Philadelphia: American College of Physicians, 2003]. N Engl J Med 2003;349(19): 1878).

Comparison to a Classic or Standard in the Field

Every field in medicine has two or three standard reference books, such as Harrison's *Principles of Internal Medicine* or Nelson's *Pediatrics*. If and when a new book is published to challenge the champion, it is only fair that the reviewer make a comparison of the two.

The Biopsy of Favorite Topics
One approach to assessing the value of a book is to look up your favorite topic, for example, headache, myocardial infarction, breast cancer, or myositis ossificans. Is the topic covered in the book? If so, is the information complete and timely? In your review tell the reader what you found.

An example of the biopsy approach appears in the *Croatian Medical Journal*. The review discusses one of my favorite books, a catalog of etymologic origins of medical words. The review says a little about the book, and then goes on to give an example for each letter of the alphabet from "A" ("ARTERY is a derivation of a Greek word for an air duct . . . ") to Z ("ZYGOMATIC was taken from the Greek *zygon*, 'a yoke or crossbar by which two draft animals can be hitched to a plow or wagon'") (Marusiae A. Review of: Haubrich WS. Medical meanings: a glossary of word origins [Philadelphia: American College of Physicians, 1997]. Croat Med J 1999;40(1):38–39).

On a more practical level, if I were reviewing a comprehensive reference on obstetrics, I might check how the author(s) handle placenta previa or antibiotic use during pregnancy. In a pediatrics text, I might check current immunization recommendations, since they change a little from year to year.

Overview with Criticism: Balancing Good Features with Problems
In a review of a 219-page book about breast cancer, the reviewer states, "*Prognostic and Predictive Factors in Breast Cancer* is a well-written, compact reference book." On balance, he goes on to observe, "The biggest problem with a book that attempts to review fast-moving fields such as breast cancer is that by the time it is published, some material is obsolete and the newest areas are not covered. For instance, this book has no discussion of sentinel-node analysis and clinical trials of trastuzumab, which were still in progress when it was written" (Rimm D. Review of Walker RA. Prognostic and predictive factors in breast cancer [New York: Martin Dunitz, 2003]. N Engl J Med 2004;350(2):200–201).

How to Write the Book Review

In broad terms, different types of book are reviewed differently. If the book is a text, intended for students, clarity is most important and the occasional minor error is less important. What is crucial is the book's ability to provide the student with concepts and templates that can aid in future learning.

The medical reference book is a different story. Here the book reviewer must assess the factual accuracy of the book. As Day[6] states, "Any professional librarian will tell you that an inaccurate reference book is worse than none at all." Clinical decisions will be made based on what is in the pages. It seems melodramatic to say that a factual error on the page could kill a patient, but conceivably this could happen. (I will say more about errors in Chapter 10.)

Book reviews follow a pattern: They begin by identifying the topic of the book being reviewed, often with a verbal image that draws us in to read further. Then comes the analysis of the work, including good points and any deficiencies. Finally there is the summary, including who might want to read this book.

Beginning the Review

Since book reviews should not be too long, it is a good idea to start the first paragraph by identifying the book being reviewed and probably giving a strong hint of your overall assessment. Here is a textbook example: "Cohn and Edmunds have edited exactly the kind of state-of-the-art textbook that is essential for practitioners and students of cardiac surgery" (Rosengart TK. Review of Cohn LH, Edmunds LH. Cardiac surgery in the adult. 2nd ed. [New York: McGraw-Hill, 2003]. N Engl J Med 2004;350:1162).

With a little more flair: "*Black Lung* is a scholarly work, a grim story, grimly told" (Cameron IA. Review of: Derickson A. Black lung: anatomy of a public health disaster [Ithaca, NY: Cornell University Press, 1998]. The Pharos 2002;65(3):50).

In a review of an edited book about health care reform, the reviewer begins, "The failure of President Clinton's health reform plan in 1994 was followed by multiple efforts at market-driven reform in the US health services system. This book is about those efforts" (Anderson R. Review of: Bloche MG, ed. The privatization of health care reform: legal and regulatory perspectives [New York: Oxford University Press, 2003]. JAMA 2004;291:375).

One enthusiastic reader begins by stating, "I really liked this book" (Neelon FA. Review of: Bittersweet: diabetes, insulin and the transformation of illness [Chapel Hill, NC: University of North Carolina Press, 2003]. JAMA 2004;291:745).

Good Points and Bad

This section, the body of the review, answers these questions: What did I like about the book? What could the author have done better?

Here is one example of the counterpoint. In discussing a book about "giving news" in both everyday talk and clinical settings, the reviewer offers praise: "Readers will come to understand the sequential steps that make up 'giving news,' just what makes information into news, and the different sequences we use to deliver good news and bad." On balance the reviewer continues, "However, the reader not already familiar with linguistic terms may find the book's terminology a bit over-technical" (Platt FW. Review of: Bad news, good news: conversational order in everyday talk and clinical settings [Chicago: University of Chicago Press, 2003]. JAMA 2003;290:3256).

One more example, from a review on American colonial medicine: On the plus side, the reviewer states, "*Medicine in Colonial America* is chockablock with detail presented in a clear writing style, covering a large territory in easy fashion—a good introduction to the novice." And yet, on the other hand, "There are a few errors. Samuel Johnson is misidentified as Ben Johnson" (Murray TJ. Review of: Reiss O. Medicine in colonial America [Lanham, MD: University Press of America, 2000]. The Pharos 2002;65(2):41–42).

Once as I was basking in the glow of a uniformly favorable review of one of my early books, my editor and mentor commented, "A review without a single criticism of the book lacks credibility."

When you are writing a book review, the body of the review should answer many of the questions listed in Table 7.1.

TABLE 7.1. Questions for the book reviewer

Is the book's topic important?
Is the information timely?
Is the content appropriate for the intended audience?
Is the book appropriately organized?
Is the writing clear?
Is the style consistent throughout the book?
Is my favorite topic covered appropriately?
Has the author included appropriate tables and figures?
Are there misspellings and minor errors?
Are there significant errors of fact?
Is the index adequate to find what I want to find?
Are the paper and binding of good quality?
Is the book worth the cost?
Do you recommend the book and, if so, for which readers?

The Reviewer's Conclusion

In the end, the reviewer should summarize his or her opinion of the book, and which readers are likely to find it useful. In the review of the book *Prognostic and Predictive Factors in Breast Cancer* cited above, the reviewer ends by stating that it "will be a valuable addition to libraries, especially at teaching institutions" (Rimm D. Review of Walker RA. Prognostic and predictive factors in breast cancer [New York: Martin Dunitz, 2003]. N Engl J Med 2004;350(2):200–201). The publisher may not be overjoyed by this summary, since libraries at teaching institutions are a very small market. For a book to be successful, it must appeal to a larger market, generally of practicing clinicians.

Contrast this summary with a review of a popular medical dictionary, "All in all, this book contains an extraordinary amount of authoritative information between its covers, and at that, for a price per pound considerably less than that for fresh Alaska salmon. Every doctor's office and hospital nursing station should have one" (Fortuine R. Review of Dorland's illustrated medical dictionary, 30th ed. [Philadelphia: WB Saunders, 2003]. JAMA 2003;290(24):3255–3256).

Without your personal opinion, your earlier comments are less helpful to your reader.

What Makes an Excellent Book Review and What Does Not

The excellent book review is informative and brightly written. It must offer a personal judgment of the merits of the book. But the review must not be too clever. In writing the book review, there is a great tendency for the reviewer to attempt to outshine the author.

The review of *Dorland's Medical Dictionary* mentioned above begins by providing some new information. I enjoyed learning the following: "Who uses a medical dictionary? It may surprise some that physicians are probably not the principal users, but rather medical students, other health care professionals, medical transcriptionists, and perhaps even lawyers and journalists."

I felt compelled to read the review that began, "Have you ever wondered, after a hard week at work, why you decided to become a doctor? If so, you might want to read this book" (McClure I. Review of: Baiev K. The oath: a surgeon under fire [New York: Simon and Schuster, 2003]. BMJ 2004;328:354).

Sometimes the review walks a fine line between writing vividly and being too clever. In reviewing a book that presents arguments against evolutionary psychology, the reviewer begins, "The contributors to the volume—an eclectic mix of biologists, sociologists, and philosophers—evidently feel about evolutionary psychology the way I feel about squirrels who steal food from the bird feeders in my backyard" (Perlman R. Review of: Rose H, Rose S, eds. Alas, poor Darwin: arguments against evolutionary psychology [New York: Harmony Books, 2000]. The Pharos 2002;65(3):48–49).

And sometimes, the reviewer is too witty for my taste. The following is the first sentence in a review of a book on alternative medicine in America: "Medical doctors and naturopaths work together to manage the publicly-funded King County Natural Medicine Clinic in Seattle. Is this a manifestation of Northwestern coffee intoxication?" (Zaroff L. Review of: Whorton JC. Nature cure: the history of alternative medicine in America [New York: Oxford University Press, 2002]. The Pharos 2003;66(4):38–39).

Yes, I am well aware of the irony that I am reviewing the writing of reviewers. And I am doing so without offering them an opportunity for rebuttal.

Cautions When Writing a Book Review

I have at times been asked to review a book that might be perceived to compete with one of my own books. For example, I edit a book used in medical school clinical clerkships. If I am sent a clerkship book written or edited by another person, I will decline to review this book. There would be a genuine conflict of interest. This, of course, means that during the publication life of *The Clinician's Guide to Medical Writing* I cannot review any books on medical writing.

The second caution concerns personal relationships. Criticizing an author's book in print is like striking someone's child. The negative comments can be taken very personally. If you are asked to review a book written or edited by a colleague who is a personal acquaintance, I suggest that you pass the opportunity to someone else. Declining the review helps assure an unbiased evaluation of the book, and it can prevent the loss of a friend.

OTHER MEDICAL PUBLICATION MODELS

There are other medical publication opportunities. If you have a special interest, such as poetry or medical history, you might want to consider one of the following. I have listed some journals as examples; I am confident that the models described are found in a variety of journals. If you aspire to write in any of these models, be sure to first identify your target publication, and prepare your submission so that it looks like those that have been published.

Poetry

JAMA publishes a regular column titled "Poetry in Medicine." Some other journals do also. Some recently published JAMA poems have been titled "Deep Structures," "Evening Ice

Cream," and "Brine." Brine begins:

> I am swimming across a large pool of brine
> Clawing my way through dense algae ...
> > (*Straus MJ. Brine. JAMA 2004;291:405.*)

About My Practice

Each edition of *American Family Physician* has a column "Diary from a Week in Practice." Physicians discuss specific patient encounters and their significance. Here is an abbreviated excerpt from a recent column: "When I was a medical student, I stood in awe of my confident, decisive physician-teachers. How did they arrive at such self-assuredness? I think of them today when Mrs. M, a 74-year-old woman with hypertension who's always running out of medications, says: 'I've been short of breath for two weeks.' Her symptoms come on when walking, which also gives her calf pain ..." (Gross P. Diary from a week in practice. Am Fam Physician 2004;69 (2):295–296).

Cortlandt Forum has short vignettes written by doctors titled, "My Most Memorable Patient."

History of Medicine

Some journals publish articles about medical history, a favorite topic of many clinicians. For example, in writing about the Civil War, Bollet states, "Supplying armies with fresh vegetables to prevent scurvy was always difficult, even for the tiny, 15,000 man, pre-Civil War United States army. Scurvy was the most common disease reported from frontier posts ..." (Bollet AJ. Malnutrition in civil war armies. The Pharos 2003;66(4);19–28).

X-ray or Photo Quiz

Consultant presents a continuing section, "Photo Quiz." Here authors supply photographs or radiographs accompanied by brief medical histories. The challenge to the clinician is to identify the diagnosis, which is presented later in the journal.

Movie Reviews

The Pharos publishes outstanding movie reviews. In a review of *A Beautiful Mind*, the reviewer writes, "For those who say that I never praise a picture, get ready to eat your words. *A Beautiful Mind* respects the viewer's intelligence, is entertaining, and, wonder of wonders, has a beginning, a middle and an end. The film's cohesion is undoubtedly due to the scenes having been filmed sequentially, an unusual occurrence in Hollywood today" (Dans PE. Review of: A beautiful mind (movie). The Pharos 2002;65(2):32–33).

A movie review column in a journal tends to be written by the same person each month. However, if you wish to undertake the task, there is no reason that you could not suggest such a column to your favorite specialty journal if none already exists.

Curbside Consults

An ongoing feature of *Postgraduate Medicine* is the "Curbside Consult" section. Questions are posed by practicing clinicians, with answers by experts in the field. In a recent issue, a Texas physician asked whether immunization with pneumococcal vaccine could prevent bacterial sinusitis caused by *Streptococcus pneumoniae*. The answer was that no such reduction has been demonstrated (Curbside consults. Postgrad Med 2004; 115(1):33–34).

A Piece of My Mind

"A Piece of My Mind" is the title of a feature in JAMA. Similar columns appear in many other publications, offering you the opportunity to write about something that is on your mind. Topics that are fair game are insights from an encounter with a patient, thoughts about the future of medicine, or reflections on how your profession affects you as a person.

In a recent column, the author wrote about wearing a white coat: "What is it about the physician's white coat that differentiates it from the ones worn by the Good Humor man or Benny Goodman at the bandstand?" (Hostetter MK. Stitches. JAMA 2004;291(3):282).

One of the best features of this publication model is that it is egalitarian. Publication is open to all, not just to members of prestigious academic departments. What is submitted is judged solely on its merits—the impact of the message and the clarity of the writing.

Practice Tips

In *Emergency Medicine* the column is titled "Tricks of the Trade"; in *Consultant*, look for "Practical Pointers." In practice tips columns, clinicians share ways to make practice more efficient and enjoyable. Long ago, I contributed a tip on how to administer eyedrops to a squirming infant who won't open the eyes. (Do so by holding the infant face up. Administer two to three eyedrops to the inner canthus of the eye, even with the eyes tightly closed. Eventually the infant opens the eyes and then the drops enter the eyes.)

In *Consultant*, William J. Herbert, DO, of Hermitage, Pennsylvania, advocates covering gynecologic stirrups with seasonally appropriate socks that have patterns such as hearts (for Valentine's day), Christmas motifs, or shamrocks (Herbert WJ. Practical pointers. Consultant 2003; 43(14): 1661).

Newspaper Column

Some physicians write a column for a local newspaper or send out a monthly newsletter from their practices. In a letter published in *Medical Economics*, one clinician writes: "For the past year, I've used a technique that has generated one or two new-patient visits a week. I write a column called 'A Doctor Speaks from the Heart' for the monthly newsletter of a large retirement community that's located near my practice" (Hoenig LJ. Letter. Med Econ 2004;81(1):13).

Topics that might be discussed in a newspaper column or newsletter include:

- When to call the doctor if a child is sick
- Who should get a flu shot
- First aid for acute injuries

■ How to buy medicine at the lowest cost
■ Danger signs in common illnesses
■ How to prevent falls in the elderly
■ Thoughts about herbal remedies
■ Tort reform and access to care

You and I could develop a long list of topics. The key is to keep the contributions short and memorable. Also, be sure to avoid medical jargon when writing for the public. When you undertake to write a column, you are agreeing to produce a written work at regular intervals, and hence the obligation should not be undertaken lightly. However, clinicians who write for the public enjoy the rewards of having readers in their communities remark, "I liked your article in the newspaper this week."

REFERENCES

1. Jordan EP, Shepard WC. Rx for medical writing. Philadelphia: WB Saunders; 1952:32.
2. Onions CT. The Oxford dictionary of English etymology. Oxford, England: Oxford University Press; 1979:301.
3. Huth EJ. Writing and publishing in medicine. 3rd ed. Baltimore: Williams & Wilkins; 1999:112.
4. LaVigne P. Letters to the editor. In: Taylor RB, Munning KA, eds. Written communication in family medicine. New York: Springer-Verlag; 1984:50.
5. Journal of the American Medical Association. Instructions for Authors. Available at: http://jama.ama-assn.org/inora_current/dtl.
6. Day RA. How to write and publish a scientific paper. 5th ed. Westport, CT: Oryx; 1998:176.

8

Writing Book Chapters and Books

Writing and editing medical books and chapters can be a lot of fun. This activity can also be immensely frustrating, as you will learn as we go along in this chapter. In the spirit of full disclosure, over the past 30+ years I have edited 18 medical reference books and have authored four books for clinicians and five trade books, and contributed dozens of book chapters to the books of various editors.

First, I will discuss medical books in general. Medical books can be categorized in several ways. One classification is by use: When thinking about medical books by use, we can identify *textbooks,* which are intended to be used by students as part of a course or clerkship; *reference books,* used to look up information; and what I call *enrichment books,* intended to be read for pleasure and personal growth. My textbook *Fundamentals of Family Medicine* is familiar to many medical students (Taylor RB, ed. Fundamentals of Family Medicine, 3rd ed. New York: Springer-Verlag, 2003). It contains 27 clinical chapters linked by case discussions that all involve members of a large, multigenerational family plus questions for class discussion. Dambro's *5-Minute Clinical Consult* (published annually by Lippincott Williams & Wilkins) is one of many broad-based medical reference books; I doubt that anyone other than the editor has ever read it cover to cover. *Stories of Sickness* (Brody H. Stories of Sickness. New Haven, CT: Yale University Press, 1987), an enrichment book written by a philosopher–physician, describes the patient's narration of the experience of sickness as an essential part of the act of healing. Enrichment books can be written for a medical audience, for the so-called lay audience, or both. Books written specifically for the lay audience are called trade books.

Looking at books another way, there are *edited books* and *authored books.* Edited books contain the works of two or more *contributors* not listed on the cover. With many chapters, often written by several coauthors, large reference books in major medical specialties may have several hundred contributors. If you count the contributors to your own subspecialty's leading reference book, I would be surprised if the total is less than 50, and it is probably over 100 for the largest specialties. Hence, edited books are identified by the name of the editor, or, in the case of a book with many editors, by the editor-in-chief. Edited books may take one of several forms: A true edited reference book has almost certainly been read and actually edited by the persons named on the cover. An anthology or conference proceedings may be compiled without the editor having much ability to edit content or coordinate styles.

Authored books are written by a single author or perhaps a small team. All names are on the cover as authors. This book is an authored book, written by me. As a broad generality, edited books are more likely to cover a wide spectrum of topics and be larger volumes. Authored books are most likely to be smaller and more focused.

Authored books are usually specialized. As described by LaVigne:[1] "A specialized book, also known as a technical publication, monograph, or scholarly work, is distinguished by the sophisticated level of its content. Since the specialized book is written for an author's colleagues and peers, it does not need to be as comprehensive as a text on the topic, nor as comprehensible as a book written for the general public."

When all the above is considered, your entry into book publishing is most likely to come as an invitation to contribute a chapter to an edited reference book.

BOOK CHAPTERS

The invitation to write a book chapter is flattering and, as one who has extended many such invitations, I know that most invitees say, "Yes." As a clinician, you are most likely to be invited to write a book chapter if you have a special practice-based interest that you have described in print. This may be considered one of the benefits of writing review articles. Let's say that your special interest is the evaluation of chest pain. You have published several review articles in controlled-circulation medical journals discussing the possible causes of chest pain, the different types of angina pectoris, and the causes of noncardiac chest pain. About this time, imagine the plight of a reference book editor whose favorite author on chest pain has already agreed to write on this topic for the compiler of a competing book. In searching for a replacement, the editor comes across your articles and sends you a letter or an e-mail message. You are on your way to being a book chapter author.

Occasionally an editor needs a chapter on a topic that is rarely covered or an emerging issue on which few have written. In such instances, the volume editor may look for an author who writes on a variety of topics, and invite this clinician to take on the "hard to place" topic. In planning the edited reference book *Difficult Diagnosis* (Philadelphia: WB Saunders, 1985), I decided to have a chapter on hyperhidrosis—excessive sweating. I found no experts that had claimed that topic, and so I asked a generalist colleague if she would be willing to take it on. She agreed, and contributed an excellent chapter.

The Invitation to Write a Book Chapter

You feel honored to be selected as a potential author. You are grateful, thrilled, and energized. You want to call today and accept before the editor has a change of heart. But wait. There are some issues to be considered.

One of the issues you need not be concerned about is how much you will be paid for your chapter. In almost all instances, the answer is "nothing." Although it would be theoretically fair to allocate royalties among the contributing authors of a book, the accounting realities would be overwhelming, and the dollar amounts tiny. Instead, you will (almost certainly) receive a copy of the finished book, an entry on your curriculum vitae, and the editor's endless gratitude.

For the academician, a book chapter invitation presents an important career advancement issue. The greatest academic rewards come from the publication of reports of original research (see Chapter 9). In the hierarchy of publications that can support a bid for promotion to senior faculty status, book chapters are in the middle of the list, below the meta-analysis and definitive literature review published in a peer-reviewed journal and above a letter to the editor and book review.

For the clinician, writing a book chapter on your special clinical topic—for example, the treatment of resistant psoriasis or radioactive implant therapy of prostate cancer—can help establish your national reputation and thereby obtain referrals from clinicians who agree with what is in your chapter.

About the Agreement to Write a Chapter

Before accepting the book chapter invitation, there are several questions to ask. These are listed in Table 8.1. I clearly would not accept the invitation to write a chapter unless the editor had a contract with a publisher; I might agree to write contingent upon the editor obtaining a contract, but I would not begin work until publication is assured. Once you are sure that a book contract exists, I consider the two most important questions on the list to be those that concern the page allocation and the chapter deadline. Before beginning to write you must have these numbers clearly in mind. It is all too easy to write a book chapter that is much too long, and that then needs to be cut; this represents wasted effort for both you and the editor.

TABLE 8.1. Questions to ask the volume editor when invited to contribute a chapter to an edited book

Who is going to publish the book, and do you have a signed contract?
What other books have you edited and who has published them?
May I review a full table of contents or topic outline, to see what others will cover?
Who will be some of the other authors in the book?
What will be the topic of my chapter?
Is there a special way you, as editor, want the topic handled?
What is the space allocation for my chapter (stated in double-spaced manuscript pages)?
What is the deadline for manuscript submission?
May I engage one or more coauthors?
Will I receive payment for my chapter?
Will I receive a copy of the finished book?

The deadline is especially important because the editor must receive all manuscripts at about the same time, review them promptly, and get them all in print before the clinical recommendations go out of date. One or two tardy chapters can, and sometimes do, hold up production of a book, ultimately compromising its usefulness (and sales). Or, there is another possibility. Two years ago, my wife and I cruised on the Norwegian Coastal Lines; ours was a working cargo and ferryboat that stopped at more than 40 ports as we sailed down the coast of Norway. Stops at ports of call might be 30 minutes or two hours. The captain warned us sternly on the first day, "There are no late passengers. There are only passengers who have been left behind." The editor may decide that your chapter can be "left behind" and go to print without your contribution. This happens.

What is Negotiable?
An agreement to write a book chapter has explicit and implicit commitments from you and the book editor. You may be startled to note the casual agreement between you and the compiler, sometimes only a verbal commitment on the telephone. At some later time, the publisher will send you a more formal agreement, which has at its core that the copyright to your chapter will be assigned to the publisher.

I advise not being concerned about this copyright assignment. First, it is standard in the trade and is not negotiable. Second, it rarely presents a problem. The only consideration arises when you have an innovative figure, table, mnemonic, or similar entity in your chapter, and you are sure that you will want to use this item in the future. In this case, you may be able to get the publisher to agree that the specific item is included in your chapter for "one-time use." If such agreement is not possible and you still wish the chapter published, you should have no problem using your innovative figure or table in later work, but you will need to request permission from the book's publisher for such use. Obtaining permission under such circumstances is usually quite easy.

Table 8.2 lists items that you may or may not be able to negotiate when invited to write a book chapter.

TABLE 8.2. Writing a book chapter: what is negotiable and what is not

---

Possibly negotiable:
  Exact title of the chapter
  Inviting coauthors
  How the topic will be handled
  Headings in the chapter
  Paying for artwork and permissions
  Future use of a specific figure or other item in the chapter without permission
  from the publisher

Probably not negotiable:
  Topic of your chapter
  Deadline for manuscript submission
  Payment for the chapter

Definitely not negotiable:
  Copyright assignment
  Future use of all chapter content without permission from the publisher

---

Preparing and Submitting Your Chapter

Writing a book chapter is much like writing a review article, which I described in Chapter 6. They are similar in that you must begin with a limited topic, decide on a concept and structure for what you want to say, do careful research and select references carefully, write a well-organized and authoritative essay, and then summarize while staying within appropriate page limits. But there are differences: The topic is likely to be assigned, the structure and headings may be assigned, a specific feature such as an algorithm may be required, coordination with other contributors may be needed to avoid overlap, and the deadline may be quite firm to assure timely publication. An example follows.

Earlier in this chapter I mentioned the multiauthor reference book *Difficult Diagnosis*. This book presented the diagnostic approach to a selected group of challenging problems with "enigmatic clinical presentations." Examples included fever of unknown origin, jaundice, and pelvic pain in women. Contributors were invited from many specialties. In planning the book, I decided that each chapter should have the same six major headings: Background, including definitions, incidence of the problem, and a laundry list of possible causes; History, to include what I called "high-payoff questions";

Physical Examination, including the significance of key findings; Diagnostic Studies, including laboratory investigations, diagnostic imaging, and other tests; Assessment, to include a diagnostic algorithm; and References, but no more than 25 citations. Therapy was not to be covered unless integral to diagnosis, such as the sometimes helpful response of gout to colchicine. I even wrote a sample chapter, "Acute Headache," and sent a copy to all authors recruited. The authors were seasoned clinicians and distinguished academicians.

Months later, when chapters were submitted, most authors had followed directions. They used my headings, provided laundry lists of possible causes of dysphagia and hypocalcemia that I still use today, identified high-payoff questions, and constructed useful algorithms. Only a few authors went their own way with different headings and varying concepts to their chapters. When the nonconforming chapters didn't seem to fit, the authors and I negotiated. When the "different drummer" concept seemed to fit the topic better than my prescribed headings, no change was recommended.

In the end, I believe that the contributors and I created a great book. It has innovative features and covers a special group of challenging medical topics. I relate all this because I believe that the success of the book can be attributed to the hard work and skill of authors who, for the most part, followed instructions that called for them to unify headings, limit reference citations, and construct some items—lists of possible causes, high-payoff questions, and algorithms—that readers can find in (almost) every chapter.

Chapter Structure

As noted above, the book editor may be quite specific about concept and headings, or you may be allowed to develop your own approach. The latter is more common, and most book editors do not prescribe structure as precisely as I did with *Difficult Diagnosis*.

As part of a compiled work, Joseph E. Scherger, M.D., and I wrote a chapter, on "Writing a Medical Article."[2] Our topic, as implicit in the title, was on how to write a medical article, and our approach was based on a workshop that we had presented several times. We approached the chapter as a series of 10 steps, with suggested time allocations which now, years later, I believe were not long enough.

1. Conceptualize the subject of the article (1–3 days)
2. Review the literature (1–2 weeks)
3. Select the appropriate readership and journal (1 day)
4. Organize and outline the content of the article (1 week)
5. Select a title (1 day)
6. Write the first draft (1–2 weeks)
7. Write the first revision (1 week)
8. Submit the manuscript for review by selected colleagues (1–2 weeks)
9. Write a final draft (1–3 weeks)
10. Submit the paper for publication (1 day)

Organizing a book chapter or review paper along the lines of these 10 steps is a handy method of creating structures. In other cases, the chapter's structure and headings will evolve from the topic. David B. Nash, M.D., asked me to write a chapter for an edited "enrichment" book about the future of medical practice. My chapter assignment was "The Future of Primary Care and Family Practice" (Taylor RB. The future of primary care and family practice. In: Nash DB. Future practice alternatives in medicine. New York: Igaku-Shoin, 1987: 265–300). I was given a flexible page limit, a deadline, and free rein. After much thought, I devised the following major headings for what became a very long, 35-page chapter:

What Is Primary Care?	Starting with a definition is classic.
Current Health Issues	What's going on that makes a difference?
Forces Shaping Primary Care	Issues specific to the topic are here.
Trends in Primary Care	So, what's happening now?
Family Practice as a Prototype of Primary Care	The chapter title implied a focus on family practice.
Emerging Controversies Among Specialties	Some issues are arising.

Growth Areas in Primary Care	Geriatrics, sports medicine, occupational medicine, and more.
Practice Opportunities in Primary Care	Where the jobs are and will be in the future.
Survival Skills for Primary Care Physicians	Beginning with: Respond to patient needs.
What's Ahead in Medicine	Predicting the future (this is a bad idea).

In this chapter, looking back, I constructed some very nice tables, such as the one listing the characteristics of primary, secondary, and tertiary medical care (Table 10.2 in the book). On balance, I think I tried to cover too much, with 10 major headings as evidence. And writers should not predict the future in writing, unless forecasting trends or events is the topic of the paper.

If asked to write a chapter on a clinical topic, such as gastroesophageal reflux disease or incontinence in the elderly, keep in mind that the classic headings for a clinical chapter in a medical reference book are going to be very similar to those in the *Difficult Diagnosis* book, with treatment added. Or you may think of your clinical SOAP note: Subjective, Objective, Assessment, and Plan. With a few additions, such as epidemiology, SOAP is a useful concept for a clinical chapter. If asked to write on a disease topic and given no other instructions, think about the topics in Table 8.3.

Submitting Your Book Chapter
This should be the easy part. Do your best to make it so. If you have carefully followed the editor and publisher's instructions, and have completed your chapter on time, submission should be a breeze. Verify that you have not exceeded your page allocation. Read it through one last time to find the instance in which you have repeated or contradicted yourself. Then, to be sure that you have not forgotten anything, review the checklist in Table 10.2 before sending your chapter to the editor.

How you actually submit your chapter will vary with the book editor and publisher. For my last two edited books, all

TABLE 8.3. Classic headings in book chapters on medical diseases

Definition
Epidemiology
Etiology/pathogenesis
Clinical features
Diagnosis, including history, physical examination, and diagnostic tests
Treatment
Prognosis
Prevention

manuscripts were submitted online, with only original art arriving by mail. Your role, as a contributor, is to submit your manuscript as requested by the editor.

EDITED BOOKS

In the area where I lived in upstate New York, people had a saying: If you hire six carpenters to do a job, only two will show up; one will have a sore back and the other one will have to go home to get his tools. There is an analogous saying in medical publishing: If you, as a compiling editor, contract with three authors to contribute chapters and then seek the chapters at deadline time, one will be months behind on commitments that come before your book, one will be on a year-long sabbatical in a remote village overseas, and one will have forgotten about the project entirely.*

You as the Initiator of an Edited Book

The initiator of an edited book should have certain characteristics: You should have a fair amount of experience as a book chapter contributor. It would be good to have a name that is well known among potential contributors, but this is not a requirement if you have a very good idea and a signed contract. You must be willing to spend nights and weekends

* If my memory is correct, I read this tale of three authors in the preface to a book published about 15 to 20 years ago. I cannot recall the name of the author or book and, to help me avoid accidental plagiarism, I would be grateful if a reader could supply this information for the next edition of *The Clinician's Guide to Medical Writing*.

on the project, especially when chapter manuscripts arrive, since they are all going out of date as they sit on your desk. You must be tactful, since you will be dealing with some colossal egos, as a few contributors decide they know better than you how the book should be compiled. And you must be tenacious, since the worst thing you can do in an edited book is let the project die. This death can occur when half the chapters are in hand, and the authors of the other half are behaving like the apocryphal three authors described above.

Planning an Edited Book

There are major edited books (such as *Harrison's Principles of Internal Medicine*) and there are focused books (such as *Written Communication in Family Medicine*, cited above). In most areas of medicine, there really is no room for another major edited book. The issue is not that you could not produce a big book that is better than those available; the truth is that the publisher cannot afford the financial risk of failure inherent in adding a new expensive product to a crowded market.

If planning an edited book, think about a focused product. The traditional approach is to marry a group of health problems to an age group, gender, geographic location, or medical specialty. Currently there are books on dermatologic diseases of children, medication use during pregnancy, and geriatric neuropsychiatry. There have been books about gynecologic, behavioral, or musculoskeletal problems in primary care. I await the inevitable publication of *Maternity Care of the Geriatric Patient, Sports Injuries During Labor and Delivery,* and *Pediatric Alzheimer's Disease.*

An early decision in planning an edited book on health problems is as follows: Do I want to present my chapters as diagnoses (such as myocardial infarction) or as clinical presentations, that is, symptoms or signs (such as chest pain)? Most medical books choose the former. It is handy and traditional. However, patients present to clinicians with symptoms and signs, not diagnoses, which speaks to the utility of presentation-structured books like *Difficult Diagnosis*. As a hint in recruiting authors, it is much easier to recruit authors to write on diseases than on signs or symptoms. Physicians like to take ownership of a disease, and will write endlessly to hold on to their turf. On the other hand, few clinicians claim expertise, much less ownership, of clinical presentations such as cyanosis, hemoptysis, or, as mentioned earlier, hyperhidrosis.

At a minimum, you will need to plan the following for your new edited book:

- Compelling reason for the book
- A good idea of who will buy the book
- Overall length of the book
- Number and titles of the chapters
- Short description of what should be included in each chapter
- A list of potential authors
- The time and commitment you will need to complete the project

How much time commitment will be needed? Compiling an edited medical book is a 2-year commitment—if all goes well. The good news is that you will not be working overtime for the full 24 months. Editing a book occurs in phases requiring intense effort, alternating with times when the editor has little to do. After a contract has been signed, there are three major phases when evening and weekend effort will be needed. Phase one is author recruitment. Contacting and reaching agreement with all the book's primary authors will take a lot of work, as described below. After all authors are recruited, things are quiet while authors write; at least you hope they are writing. Phase two comes when all the manuscripts arrive. The manuscript editing time is the busiest of all, because of the need to verify many facts and to negotiate changes with contributors. Phase three is proofreading, which cannot be delegated to others. Each contributor should proofread his or her own contribution. In my experience, however, most chapter authors are dismal proofreaders and you, as editor, must take responsibility for all errors by checking every word carefully.

The first step, after planning and committing yourself to your edited book, is getting a contract with a publisher. This is accomplished by submitting a proposal.

The Book Proposal and Contract

What follows regarding book proposals and contracts applies to both edited and authored books.

Finding the Right Person

Not long after deciding upon the much-needed edited book you will compile, you must find a publisher. And at that publishing company you must find the "acquisitions editor," the person who can actually negotiate a contract (with approval from the publisher, the person who controls the company budget). To locate the right publisher, look for one who publishes in your field. Some publishers bring out a number of radiology and plastic surgery books, those with many illustrations and requiring specialized production. Some publishers prefer primary care books. Another publisher may specialize, to some degree, in psychiatry and psychology books. Check the books on your own bookshelf to see who is publishing in your specialty. Visit individual publisher Web sites or Amazon.com, or go to the Literary Market Place (http://www.literarymarkeplace.com) to see who publishes what type of books.

After you have identified one or two potential publishers for your book, find the acquisitions editor in one of two ways. If you are going to a major medical meeting in your specialty, visit the exhibit booths of the publishers you are targeting. At the booth, you will find salespeople, but also at the meeting may be an acquisitions editor. Ask the salesperson whether the acquisitions editor is at the meeting and, if so, when he or she will return to the booth so that you can discuss your idea. This approach takes some effort and a little serendipity, but nothing replaces face-to-face contact.

Plan B, if you cannot meet in person, is to use the telephone and network research to track down the acquisitions editor. Let's imagine that you are a radiologist, and that you have a great idea for a new book in diagnostic imaging. Your research has shown that XYZ Publishers has a very good list of radiology books. Call the company and ask to speak to the acquisitions editor for medical radiology books. You should soon be connected with the office of the person you seek.

What's Next in Getting a Book Contract?

Tell the acquisition editor about your proposal, being sure to cover the planning topics listed above. Do not be concerned about copyright. Medical publishers are highly ethical people, and will not steal your idea. The acquisitions editor may give you some immediate feedback: "We have a book like this in production." "I don't think there is a market for this book." Or "Not a bad idea, but here is how I would modify the concept."

In most instances, your idea will be favorably received, and you will be asked to submit a proposal.

The Book Proposal

Your book proposal is a formal document. By the time it is submitted, you and your acquisitions editor may be on a first-name basis, and you may have fully discussed the proposal. You are both enthusiastic. Nevertheless, you should submit a complete, polished proposal, covering all the points listed in Table 8.4. A complete proposal, with all the pieces, is important because the next task of your acquisitions editor is to present the proposal at the regular meeting of the editors and publisher. Here is where your new editor acts as your

TABLE 8.4. What to include in a book proposal

The cover letter describing the proposed book should include the following topics:
- Title and any subtitle
- Anticipated length of the manuscript, expressed in double-spaced pages
- Number of tables and figures that will be in the book
- The book's audience, that is, who will buy the book
- The chief competing books, and how the proposed book is different
- Why you are qualified to write (or edit) the book
- Anticipated date of manuscript submission

The proposal should also include:
- A description of the book, including the intent and scope of coverage
- A table of contents
- A sample chapter, to show your style and that you can actually write
- Your curriculum vitae

Optional, but desirable, items to include:
- Expanded outline, showing headings and subheadings
- Annotated table of contents, describing the contents of each chapter

advocate to get the project approved. At this meeting, his or her most important ammunition is your proposal.

The Contract

The proposal is approved! Hooray! The standard contract is in the mail. Wonderful. But wait. Even though you receive a preprinted contract, the publisher has several "standard" contracts that can be used, according to circumstances. Some contract terms may be negotiable, and additions to the contract are possible. A review by your attorney may be helpful, but going over the contract with an experienced book author/editor is likely to be more helpful. These standard contracts are usually written in plain English, and there are really not any trick clauses. With that said, there are some key items to review carefully:

- *Royalties:* The standard was once 10% of gross sales at the U.S. retail price, and less for foreign sales. Recently publishers have learned how to cut author/editor royalties without being too obvious. The device was to change the contract to read percent of net sales. Since net sales figures are a black box impenetrable to authors, the author/editor who receives 15% of net sales may not realize that this is probably less than 10% of gross sales.
- *Advance against royalties:* Seasoned authors/volume editors should request an advance, as a warranty that the book will actually be published. Neophyte authors should ask, but are often not in a strong bargaining position even though this is really their money, and so it really isn't a cost to the publisher. You are merely getting some of your royalty payment a little early.
- *Costs related to manuscript preparation:* I always ask that the publisher pay for the cost of preparing figures and the index. These are often charged to the author, and can be an unpleasant surprise on the first royalty statement. If the book contains a lot of art and the publisher cannot agree to pay for all, ask for a grant or an allowance.
- *Author copies:* The contract will state that you get some six to 20 copies of the book. Be sure that the contract also

states that a copy will be sent to each contributor, at no cost to you.

■ *Costs related to excessive corrections on proofs:* There is nothing to be negotiated here, but be very aware of this clause. If you start rewriting on page proofs, the cost will quickly exceed your allowance for corrections, and all additional costs will be charged to your royalties.

There will be some royalty surprises. Some surprises will be bad, some good. Royalties for foreign sales are generally meager; I see no reason why this should be, but it is common. Good surprises will be unexpected, although very modest, payments when your book is translated into Spanish or Chinese. Another nice surprise is the small extra payment showing up on your royalty statement, representing your share of a fee paid by another author who has requested permission to use a table or figure in your book.

As with book chapters, copyright to the book will be owned by the publisher, a nonnegotiable item. Years from now, if and when the book is out of print, you may request that the publisher return the copyright to you, or perhaps print a new edition of the book.

Working with Authors

Your contract is signed and in the file. Your outline lists all the chapter titles. Now all you need to do is recruit a lead or primary author for each chapter. I deal with one lead author. That lead author may invite one or more coauthors, and he or she deals with the coauthors. Coauthors have their names listed on chapters, but usually do not receive copies of the book. One chapter, one book copy.

Author Recruitment

Author recruitment is a very important part of compiling an edited volume. Selecting the best contributors and communicating clearly with them can prevent hours of aggravation later.

I try to select authors who have a track record of writing, especially review articles on the same topic as the book chapter. This means that they like to write, have some talent (or a great copyeditor), and are invested in the topic. If given the choice in selecting authors, I choose reliability over brilliance every time. Enthusiasm for the project is important, and if an invitee begins to haggle over deadline dates and other items, I am likely to break off the negotiation and go on to someone else.

In extending invitations to write, I prefer to speak directly to the potential author on the telephone, especially if this is our first contact. The initial telephone discussion is then followed by a letter with a written agreement (see below). From then on, all interaction will probably be done by e-mail.

Is it difficult to recruit authors to write chapters in books? Not really. It is easiest to solicit contributors to established books—new editions of the ones everyone knows. Recruiting for a new, untested book is a little more difficult. That is why it is so important to have a publication contract before beginning recruitment. My most problematic recruitment was for the books *Difficult Diagnosis* and *Difficult Medical Management* (both published by W.B. Saunders). These were new books and they were interdisciplinary. Because of prior publications, my name is fairly well known in my specialty. But radiologists and endocrinologists are very unlikely to know me. However, I had a good concept and a signed contract with Saunders. On my first round of invitations to prospective authors in diverse specialties, my acceptance rate exceeded 60%. Why? Because I invited authors to write on their topics, largely selected by seeing who was writing review articles in controlled-circulation journals, and I believed that these clinicians would want their imprint on their topics in the new book.

Author Agreement

I have each lead author sign my own agreement form. It is probably not a legal document, and later the publisher will also send the more formal author agreement form that discusses copyright assignment. My agreement is useful when, occasionally, disagreements occur later. It anticipates the issues that may arise. My brief agreement form covers six very important topics:

- Chapter topic and title
- Page allocation
- Deadline for submission
- Coauthors are acceptable, but only one complimentary book is allocated per chapter.
- No cash payment to authors: "I hope that you will consider this invitation a great honor, especially because there is no cash payment for chapters."
- Full contact information, including e-mail address, mailing address, and all telephone numbers, including home number.

After the agreement is signed, I return a copy to the contributor and keep a copy for my files. All my agreements are with lead authors only, not with coauthors.

Author Reminders
Contributors to my edited books receive reminders about their chapters about every 6 weeks. Some are sent by mail, some by e-mail. They may discuss issues such as headings, permissions, manuscript submission, tally of how many chapters have arrived to date, and so forth. Basically they are all reminders so that my authors do not enter the "forgot about the project entirely" category.

Development Editor
You may be assigned a development editor, who will help you with issues regarding author communication and manuscript management. Some development editors are very good. In the end, however, the quality of the book will depend on your efforts and commitment.

Compiling the Book

Months ago you contracted with a number of colleagues to write chapters for your edited book. You have sent periodic reminders. Now the deadline has arrived. Will the book really come together? Will the chapters actually arrive? Will they be as good as you hope?

Fundamentally, there will be two types of problem at manuscript deadline time: One is chapters that arrive and need improvement; and the second problem is those chapters that do not arrive at all.

Editing Chapters that Arrive

Some chapter manuscripts will be better than others. Some will be perfect. After all, you have been in frequent contact with all the authors, guiding them during the writing phase. Other chapters will require editing. Here we apply the revision principles described in Chapter 3, but with a big difference. Now you are editing someone else's work, not your own. You cannot just make substantive changes; all modifications that might affect meaning must be negotiated with the author. This often means sending the chapter back and forth once or twice before you and the author agree that it is the best that it can be.

Missing Chapters

The authors of missing chapters will offer a variety of excuses. In Table 3.4 I listed some of the many reasons authors fail to complete and submit their manuscripts on time (see page 83). Of course, as volume editor, you are not really very interested in the excuse. You need a chapter manuscript.

When I plan an edited book, I create a set of three "late chapter" notices. The first begins, "This is a friendly reminder that your chapter was due three weeks ago ..." The final notice states, "This is the third and final notice that your chapter is late and is in danger of not being in the book. I know you have worked hard on this project, but the book must be submitted and published on time. Therefore, if the chapter manuscript is not on my desk by (you select the date), it will not be in the book. Packages arriving after this date will be returned unopened." By selecting authors carefully, reminding them often, and using late notices when needed, I seldom have problems with missing chapters. But occasionally it happens.

If a chapter actually does not arrive, you must face a choice. One option is to create a chapter on short notice to fill a needed gap in a book. Once while compiling a book on health promotion, I encountered an author who fooled me for weeks after the deadline. "The chapter is almost done. You will have it next week." Eventually I learned that he had done nothing, and was in no hurry to do so. The chapter was about weight control, a topic vital to a health promotion book. To fill the gap, one of the associate editors and I wrote a "weight control" chapter in about 10 days, filled the gap, and submitted an intact book manuscript. The weight control chapter was probably not the best in the book, but reviewers did not single it out for criticism (Taylor RB, Ureda JR, Denham JW. Health promotion: principles and clinical applications. Norwalk, CT: Appleton, Century Crofts, 1982).

Missing chapters force the decision, "Is this chapter expendable?" For the volume editor, the ideal edited books are those such as *Difficult Diagnosis*, which present eclectic topics, with any one expendable. In fact, in compiling such books, often with new authors in many specialties, I count on attrition of about 7% of chapters and authors. The more challenging books are those, such as a specialty textbook, that have a sequence of chapters in which no one is expendable. In this case all chapters must be received or created on short notice.

Publication of the Book

You have received all chapters, negotiated editing changes with contributors, added any appendix material, and carefully submitted everything to the publisher. Of course, you have kept a copy of everything, just in case.

Here are the steps that follow after the book is received by the publisher:

- *Verification:* An editorial assistant will check to see that everything has been received. This person will take a hard look at signed permission forms, and the publisher may refuse to go further if any permission form is missing.
- *Assignment to a production editor:* The project will be passed to a new person, the production editor. This person

has the important job of shepherding your manuscript from submission to finished book.

■ *Copyediting:* Next the manuscript will have line-by-line editing by a copyeditor who has basically two tasks. One is to fix errors of grammar and syntax without changing meaning. The second is to mark up the book for the printer, with some arcane symbols that only professional editors and printers understand.

■ *Author review of copyediting:* In many instances, the manuscript will be sent back to you and the contributors to review copyediting changes. At this stage, you will probably see some questions posed by the copyeditor, asking if this fact is true or if you really mean to say that.

■ *Marketing questionnaire:* At about this stage, the publisher's marketing department will send you a long questionnaire to complete. Questions will concern the key features of the book, the intended audience, the best figures, and so forth. Take the time to do a good job on this document, which will be the basis of the marketing program for the book.

■ *Galley proofs:* Galley proofs are your work set in print, but not divided into pages. You will review these proofs for errors and return them to the publisher. In some instances, the publisher will skip this step, especially if you have submitted a manuscript with minimal problems and if the copyeditor has asked few questions.

■ *Page proofs:* Here is your book set in pages. You will receive these for review. At this stage your job is to correct errors. That is all. This is not the time to rewrite to improve phrases or add new thoughts. Alterations at this stage are costly, and will be charged to you.

■ *Printing and binding:* This takes a while. During this time, a cover may be created, and you should ask to review the artwork. On several occasions I have picked up errors on covers for my books. In the end, the publisher will create several thousand copies of your book.

■ *Publication:* The book is released. Review copies are sent to major journals by the publisher. Copies are sent to leading book distributors.

After the Book Is Published

Now is the time to take a breather. You have your author's copy of the book in hand. It looks great. You show it to your family and friends, who may actually be impressed. You might even, as I have done for years, frame a copy of the book cover to hang on the wall of your office.

You will wait anxiously for reviews. These take a long time, as might be expected. There is a time lag at each step of mailing the review copies to the journals, assigning the book to a reviewer, and then having the reviewer submit the review, and finally experiencing the interval until publication of the review. You hope for a favorable review, remembering from Chapter 7 that a completely positive review lacks credibility.

At this time, create an errata file. As you use the book, you will find small errors, which I hope do not involve drug doses. Keep a file of these spelling glitches and minor factual misstatements, which may be correctable with the next printing.

Also, begin a file on ideas for the second edition of the book, which will come up sooner than you think. Remember that an edited book is a 2-year effort from outline to bookstore. A medical text or reference book has a useful life of about 4 years, as new knowledge makes 5-year-old books seem ancient. Your book has just been published. With a 4-year cycle, this means that you have 2 years to rest (and collect ideas) before you start work on the second edition.

Finally, as volume editor, take good care of your contributors. Send them a letter thanking them for participating. If available, include a copy of the book's reviews. Be sure that each lead author receives a copy of the book from the publisher.

THE AUTHORED BOOK

Much of what I have presented above about edited books also applies to authored books. The big difference with the authored book, of course, is that an individual or a small team undertakes to write it all.

Today not many medical reference books are written entirely by sole authors. Certainly there are no broad-based single-author medical books. Health care has become too specialized and the volume of medical knowledge is just too great for one person to cover a wide spectrum.

On the other hand, there are a number of possibilities for the aspiring book author. Many of these will be enrichment medical books. Here are some diverse examples of single-author books:

- Osler Sir W. Aequanimitas with Other Addresses. 3rd ed. Philadelphia: Blakiston, 1932. In a moment of humility, Sir William compiled an anthology of his own works. "Delivered at sundry times and in divers (sic) places in the course of a busy life, it was not without hesitation that I collected these addresses for publication."
- Major RH. Disease and Destiny. New York: Appleton-Century, 1936. Dr. Major writes of "a dominant role of disease in the destiny of the human race."
- Marti-Ibanez F. A Prelude to Medical History. New York: MD Publications, 1961. The author has compiled his lectures on medical history given to medical students at the New York Medical College.
- Brody H. Stories of Sickness. New Haven, CT: Yale University Press, 1987. Mentioned earlier in this chapter, this book describes the role of patient narrative in health care.
- Selzer R. Mortal Lessons: Notes on the Art of Surgery. New York: Touchstone, 1974. Clinicians and laypersons alike enjoyed reading about the exact location of the soul and other musings of this articulate surgeon.
- Dirckx JH. The Language of Medicine. 2nd ed. New York: Praeger, 1983. This physician presents a scholarly treatise on the evolution, structure, and dynamics of the words clinicians use.
- Maynard DW. Bad News, Good News: Conversational Order in Everyday Talk and Clinical Settings. Chicago: University of Chicago Press, 2003. The author discusses information, news, and communication in a variety of settings.
- Campo R. The Healing Art: A Doctor's Black Bag of Poetry. New York: Norton, 2003. The author discusses how poetry can help comfort and heal.

■ Feudner C. Bittersweet: Diabetes, Insulin and the Transformation of Disease. Chapel Hill, NC: University of North Carolina Press, 2003. This book chronicles the changes that have occurred in the management of a common disease.

■ Taylor RB. The Clinician's Guide to Medical Writing. New York: Springer-Verlag, 2005. Okay, so I included my own book. It *is* an authored, focused medical book.

What are the commonalities among the books listed above? They are single-author books; writing books is usually a solitary activity. They are focused, and generally appeal to clinicians with special interests in medical history, epistemology, language, alternative medicine, or other topics outside the mainstream.

Notice also that many are not published by the big conglomerate medical publishers. Such books are not big money-makers, and proposals for meritorious projects are often turned down by major publishers with the statement, "This would be a great book, but we cannot project sufficient sales to allow us to publish it." Enrichment books are more likely to be published by university presses, specialty societies, or smaller publishers that can deal with modest print runs. If you love your book and just want to see it in print, then contracting with a small publisher will not be a mistake.

If you decide to undertake an authored medical book, you will follow the same path as described in the section on edited books: Begin by clarifying your concept, and be realistic about who will buy the book. Then create a proposal packet, containing all the elements described in Table 8.4. Then find an acquisitions editor, either in person or by telephone. *Do not write the entire book* and then begin to hunt for a publisher. Editors almost always want a role in developing a book's concept and style.

Contracts for authored books differ little from those for edited books. The chief difference would be that there is no provision for copies for contributors.

The contract will specify a date when the manuscript is due. Be sure to give yourself enough time. Writing a book and doing a good job of it takes time. I suggest allowing yourself

9 to 12 months from the date of the contract. If you deliver the manuscript early, everyone will be happily surprised.

The big advantage of an authored book is that you are not dealing with egoistic contributors, and you do not need to negotiate changes with others. One disadvantage is that you are on your own, and can go off track, beginning with a good idea and then changing direction or style. While writing your book, I urge that you show consecutive chapters to your trusted colleague reviewer, asking for critical feedback.

In the end, writing a book can be exhilarating. One colleague who wrote a book during a time of major administrative challenges has said, "I wrote the book on evenings and weekends, but at the time it was the only thing keeping me sane." As I write this book, I look forward to learning what will come next in each chapter; then I write it. This is the fun of writing, especially book writing, and I hope that all readers experience the pleasure at least once in their lives.

RANDOM THOUGHTS ABOUT MEDICAL BOOKS

Professional Books and Trade Books

Professional/textbooks and trade books live in two different worlds. At the publisher's offices, there may be both text and trade divisions, but there seems to be a firewall between them.

Trade books are what general-interest (read: nonmedical) people read. Tom Clancy and J.K. Rowling write trade books. Dr. Spock's *Baby and Child Care* is a trade book. My first books, in the 1970s, were trade books, until a Harper and Row Publishers trade editor whom I never met did a remarkable thing. I had submitted a manuscript (Yes, I had written the book already, which I would not do today) about a book on symptoms and what they could mean. If an individual had heartburn, might it be gastritis, peptic ulcer disease, or stomach cancer? The trade book editor decided that the book was too technical for a lay audience. Instead of returning the manuscript to me with a form-letter rejection, he sent the book to medical editor Charles Visokay, M.D. Chuck read the manuscript, offered a contract, and Harper and Row

Medical Publishers published the book. I have been doing professional medical books ever since that time.

There are tens of thousands of trade books published every year. There are very few authors, like Tom Clancy and J.K. Rowling, who make vast sums from their royalties. Most trade authors see little income for their efforts. For that matter, neither do medical book authors earn much from their books. For clinicians, the rewards come in professional recognition, career advancement, and perhaps some patient referrals.

I believe that finding a medical publisher is much easier than finding a trade publisher. It seems that everyone in America is writing a book and seeking a publisher. Most trade publishers protect their sanity by considering submissions only through recognized literary agents. Agents, in turn, are besieged by author wannabes, and turn away almost all previously unpublished authors.

In medical publishing, there are fewer publishing companies. But there are also fewer prospective authors competing for their contracts. And to my knowledge, there are, as yet, no literary agents in medical publishing.

I much prefer the professional medical publishing milieu to the trade publishing process.

Do Not Underestimate the Effort

Editing or writing a book is a big effort. Yes, as I mentioned earlier, the intense activity comes in cycles. Nevertheless, preparing any type of book is committing your spare time to the effort. Do not undertake the job lightly. If you are planning to commit to a medical book, you must want the project a lot! I have seen clinicians come to hate the books they were working on. A few have given up midway through the project. Giving up on an authored book is bad enough. Abandoning an edited book after colleagues have worked on chapters at your request is devastating.

The Market Rules

You and your acquisitions editor must pay close attention to the question, Who will buy this book? In today's tight economic times, publishers cannot afford to ignore the market. Long ago, I wrote a short book entitled *Why Doctors Give Children Shots*. The book told the stories of communicable diseases against which we immunize children: smallpox vaccination (I mentioned that this was a very long time ago), tetanus, diphtheria, polio, and so forth. I collected some wonderful historic illustrations. It was a well-written, vividly illustrated, innovative book. There was only one small problem: Who would buy the book? The kids getting the shots were too young to read a book about medical history, however clearly written. The parents weren't especially interested in the topic, and the book was too consumer-oriented for clinicians. I made many unsuccessful efforts to find a publisher. Today the manuscript is in a cardboard box in the attic. I know how to find it, in case anyone wants to publish it.

Book Publishing and Personal Relationships

If you are interested in writing or editing medical books, I urge you to remember what I am about to write. This may be the must useful sentence in the entire chapter: *Medical book publishing is about personal relationships*. As a book editor, you work closely with your contributors. I have edited six editions of the large reference book *Family Medicine: Principles and Practice* (New York: Springer-Verlag) over 26 years. Many of my authors contributed chapters over multiple editions, and one loyal contributor has been in all six editions.

During the past three decades, I have worked with more than a dozen medical editors employed by five medical publishing houses. Medical editors usually don't fade away; they move from one medical publishing job to another. Relationships continue, and are highly valuable when you need access to an editor to evaluate a project.

Nurture your relationships with contributors and with your medical editors. Next to the exhilaration of actually writing, these can be the best part of working on medical books.

REFERENCES

1. LaVigne P. Seeking publication. In: Taylor RB, Munning KA, eds. Written communication in family medicine. New York: Springer-Verlag; 1984:57.
2. Scherger JE, Taylor RB. Writing a medical article. In: Taylor RB, Munning KA, eds. Written communication in family medicine. New York: Springer-Verlag; 1984:33–42.

9

How to Write a Report of a Clinical Study

In *The Lancet* is the report of a study that examined the risk of cancer from diagnostic x-rays, combining data from 15 developed countries (de Gonzalez AB, Darby S. Risk of cancer from diagnostic x-rays: estimates for the UK and 14 other countries. Lancet 2004;363:345–351). As an aside for those clinicians who are wondering, the conclusion is that diagnostic x-rays do contribute to cancer risk, but by only a small amount.

The *Annals of Internal Medicine* contains a report of the affect of aspirin use on the risk for colorectal cancer (Chan AT, Giovannucci EL, Schernhammer ES, et al. A prospective study of aspirin use and the risk for colorectal cancer. Ann Intern Med 2004;140(3):157–166). The conclusion is that aspirin use can reduce colorectal cancer risk; issues involved include the duration of use, the optimum dose, and the dangers of taking daily aspirin.

If you want to learn if influenza vaccine prevents acute otitis media in young children, turn to the article published in the *Journal of the American Medical Association* (JAMA) (Hoberman A, Greenberg DP, Paradise JL, et al. Effectiveness of inactivated influenza vaccine in preventing acute otitis media in young children. JAMA 2003;290:1608–1616). For the record, there were no differences between the vaccine and placebo groups.

You may be interested in knowing whether seeing the same clinician often, in contrast to seeing the "doc-of-the-day," makes a difference in health care costs. If so, read the article by Maesneer and colleagues (Maesneer JM. Provider continuity in family medicine: Does it make a difference in total health care costs? Ann Fam Med 2003;1:144–148) The answer to the question is yes. "Provider continuity with a family physician is related to lower total health care costs."

Those who want to read about a research study of surgeons swearing when operating should read the article describing what was observed when "one hundred consecutive elective operations under general anesthesia performed at a single hospital were assessed for the incidence of swearing by the operating surgeon" (Paluzzo FF, Warner OJ Surgeons swear when operating: fact or myth? BMJ 1999;319: 1611–1615.) Hint as to the outcome: "Surgeons do swear when operating, but the rate differs by specialty. Orthopaedic surgeons on average register one swear point every 29 minutes, almost twice as often as surgeons overall."

Preparing the report of original research is arguably the most challenging undertaking in medical writing. It is not necessarily that writing the report is so difficult, because the model is prescribed. In a sense, you need only fill in the blanks. The challenging part is that one needs to have a completed research study with data. What follows assumes that you have completed that task, and are composing your report for publication.

Because there is a prescribed model, writing the report of original research has an advantage over other types of medical writing. You will not need to dream up a concept and structure for the article. In previous chapters I discussed various ways to approach the review article, editorial, book chapter, and other models of medical publication. For the report of original research, there is only one model, called IMRAD. This acronym stands for the major parts of a research report: *I*ntroduction, *M*ethods, *R*esults, *a*nd *D*iscussion. The IMRAD format is what editors are accustomed to reviewing. It is what clinicians and scientists are used to reading. Deviating from this format risks summary rejection. I describe the IMRAD format below.

The rigid format for the report of original research highlights the fact that research reports are written to be published and cited, more than they are written to be read. They are intended to be repositories of scientific data rather than literary gems. They just happen to be in prose. Day[1] has summarized this viewpoint very well: "Some of my old-fashioned colleagues think that scientific papers should be literature, that the style and flair of an author should be clearly evident, and that variations in style encourage the interest of the reader. I disagree. I think scientists should indeed be interested in reading literature, and perhaps even in writing literature, but the communication of research results is a more prosaic procedure."

With that said, I still plead with authors, even those composing research papers, to construct paragraphs thoughtfully, avoid long and convoluted sentences, select words carefully, and express their ideas as clearly as possible.

THINKING ABOUT THE RESEARCH REPORT

For the clinical investigator, this is probably the most important chapter in the book, because getting research results published can be the difference between professional success and failure. It can determine whether or not one gets the big grant, or if one receives tenure. Entire academic careers have been built on a single groundbreaking research study, carefully reported in a prestigious journal. For those clinicians who are not on academic faculty and who have done a practice-based research project, remember that your research is not completed until the results are reported in print.

The five papers I cited above all had research questions that provoked my interest, and perhaps yours. I wanted to know whether diagnostic x-rays influence cancer risk, the effect of aspirin on colorectal cancer risk, whether or not influenza vaccine might reduce the incidence of middle ear infection in children, whether continuity of care really matters, and—frivolously—how much surgeons swore in the operating room. For this reason, I briefly summarized the study outcomes, even though this is a book about writing and not clinical science.

I mention the above—about my interest in the research questions that prompted the studies—because you may be tempted to stretch the definition of research too far. As a surgeon, you may consider reporting the findings of your last 200 cases of lumbar laminectomy or laparoscopic cholecystectomy. If you are an internist, you may believe that your colleagues are keenly interested in how you treated 200 consecutive patients with congestive heart failure. Such studies do not set out to answer a clinical question and do not have anything important to say. They may qualify as quality improvement efforts, but are not likely to result in a publishable research paper.

In planning a research study, I find it useful to think about how the data will be presented in print. In my mind I construct the tables I will want to use in my paper; I just don't know the numbers yet. Then I conduct the research to answer the research question and to fill in the numbers in the table.

Broadly speaking, this is the way research is properly conducted. You generate a research question, and then collect data to answer the question. "Mining" tons of data to find something, *anything*, that has statistical significance is not good research, and such a method will be evident to the informed reviewer.

When planning a research report, be aware that competition for publication space in leading refereed journals is intense, and research papers are often rewritten several times before final acceptance. Ultimately, your clinical research paper will be judged by its impact on your specialty and on the body of medical knowledge, as evidenced by its citation in other research articles, review papers, and textbooks.

THE EXPANDED IMRAD MODEL

The IMRAD model of research reports has evolved over generations of scientific publications. It has at its core four elements:

- Introduction: Why is the topic important, what prior research has been done, and what question did you set out to answer?
- Methods: Who were your subjects and what did you do to them? How did you analyze the data?
- Results: What did you find out?
- Discussion: What do your findings mean?

These four items are the core of IMRAD. Research papers, however, have more than just the four components, and I am going to present an expanded IMRAD model. Keep in mind the four key components as we explore the IMRAD and more, beginning with selection of the title for the report.

Title

Craft your title with care; it is the one part of the paper that most of your intended audience will read, and on the basis of the title, they will make decisions as to whether to read the abstract, and maybe even the rest of the paper.

The title is the "label" for the paper. The title must tell, more or less, what was studied. An early question the writer must answer is this: Should I reveal my conclusion in the title?

One of the studies cited at the beginning of the chapter is titled "Effectiveness of Inactivated Influenza Vaccine in Preventing Acute Otitis Media in Young Children: A Randomized Controlled Trial." If I read only the title, I might take away the message that flu vaccine prevents childhood ear infections. In fact, the study showed no such protection. Therefore, I believe that a better title would be "Lack of Effectiveness of Inactivated Influenza Vaccine in Preventing Acute Otitis Media in Young Children: A Randomized Controlled Trial."

Whimster[2] writes: "I believe that readers need a verb in the title, such as a newspaper headline usually has, and that to be meaningful it should convey the message, as in: 'Rickettsial endocarditis is not a rare complication of congenital heart disease in dental practice: a report of five cases.'"

Sometimes we authors like witty titles. The swearing surgeon study mentioned above ends with: "Fact or Myth?" In many cases, editors counsel against using clever phrases in titles, and rightfully so.

Note how often colons show up in article titles. They allow progression from the general to the specific, all in an integrated title phrase. See the papers cited above. One example is the title "Risk of Cancer from Diagnostic X-rays: Estimates for the UK and 14 Other Countries." The authors discuss the general problem and then the data sources. The reader has a better idea of the article's contents than if only the first phrase were listed.

On a technical basis, the instructions for authors may prescribe a word or character limit for the title. Also, I believe that titles should not contain acronyms or abbreviations, no matter how widespread the author and editor consider their use.

Authors

The chief issues in authorship of a research report are generally twofold: (1) Who is an author? (2) How shall the authors be listed?

Question 1 is clearly answered in the *Uniform Requirements for Manuscripts Submitted to Biomedical Journals*: "Authorship credit should be based only on (1) substantial contributions to conception and design, or acquisition of data, or analysis and interpretation of data; (2) drafting the article or revising it critically for important intellectual content; and (3) final approval of the version to be published. Conditions 1, 2, and 3 must all be met. Acquisition of funding, the collection of data, or general supervision of the research group, by themselves, do not justify authorship."[3]

What about adding author names of those who have contributed very little? Strasburger[4] described the problem: "Fiction is written by one individual; medical articles may be written by committee. There is no such thing as 'author inflation' in fiction, simply because there is no need for it. Medical writers must publish or perish, academically. Fiction writers must publish or perish, existentially." Despite the need to avoid perishing, it is inappropriate to have your name listed if you have not met the three criteria listed in the previous paragraph. You must not become an "author inflation" perpetrator.

No department chair or research director should insist on being named as an author unless there has been a significant contribution to the study and to writing the paper. Authorship listing by administrative fiat is academic malpractice. Adding the name of a prestigious senior faculty member as the final entry on a long author list might help get the paper a better review, but including the well-known name implies that person's active participation in the project. Gratuitous addition of an author name is not ethically appropriate.

The order in which authors are listed on the paper should be decided very early in the process, generally during one of the first meetings of the research group planning the study. Changes in the rank order can be made later if contributions of individuals to the project do not turn out to be what was originally planned.

The first author should always be the one who has done most of the work. Generally this is the person who led the research team and who has created the early drafts of the paper. From then on, authors should be listed according to how much they contributed to the study and the paper. As one whose last name begins with a letter toward the end of the alphabet, I have never considered alphabetical listings of names to be fair to the Taylors, Walshes, and Zells of the world.

A quirk of citation listing holds that when the paper is used as a reference in other studies, if your paper has seven or more authors, only the first three are named and the rest will join the et al army of obscurity.

Abstract

The abstract is an author-generated synopsis of the paper. I believe that the final version of the abstract should be the last item written, since only then will you know exactly what is in the paper that you are summarizing, and since these few paragraphs are the most read and hence the most important of the article.

In general I have always taught that the abstract should mirror the IMRAD structure of the paper. That is, the paper's introduction, methods, results, and discussion (conclusions) should each be presented in a sentence or two, and many good abstracts have exactly four short paragraphs. According to the Uniform Requirements, "The abstract should state the purposes of the study or investigation, basic procedures (selection of study subjects or laboratory animals; observational and analytic methods), main findings (giving specific data and their statistical significance if possible), and the principal conclusions. It should emphasize new and important aspects of the study or observations."[3]

The current trend is for journals to require structured abstracts.[5] This means that information in the abstract is presented according to specific headings that differ a little with each journal. Some journals prefer abstracts with full sentences; others encourage the use of phrases, such as from a report in the *British Medical Journal* (BMJ) (Cluett ER, Pickering RM, Getliffe K, Saunders NJS Randomized controlled trial of labouring in water compared with standard augmentation for management of dystocia in first stage of labor. BMJ 2004;238:314–319):

Objectives: To evaluate the impact of labouring in water during the first stage of labour on rates of epidural analgesia and operative delivery in nulliparous women with dystocia.
Design: Randomised controlled trial.
Setting: University teaching hospital in southern England.
Participants: 99 nulliparous women with dystocia (cervical dilation rate less than 1 cm/hour in active labor) at low risk of complications.

Later in the abstract, under Results and Conclusions, the style changes from phrases to complete sentences.

The instructions to authors for JAMA state, "Reports of original data should include an abstract of no more than 300 words using the following headings: Context, Objective, Design, Setting, Patients (or Participants), Interventions (include only if there are any), Main Outcome Measure(s), Results, and Conclusions. For brevity, parts of the abstract may be written as phrases rather than complete sentences."[6]

The tight word limitation and the many topics to be covered serve to get the important data into tightly written abstracts, but at the expense of some very tortuous, number-laden, and almost incomprehensible sentences in the Results section.

On a technical basis, abstracts report on work that has been done and should be written in the past tense. In the spirit of intellectual honesty, the abstract must never contain a conclusion that is not discussed in the body of the paper.

Key Words

Key words can be what keep your report from being lost in the information jungle. They are part of the retrievability process that can contribute to the number of times your paper will be cited. In the instructions to authors, many journals request that you submit three to 10 key words or short phrases. These will "assist indexers in cross-indexing the article and may be published with the abstract. Terms from the Medical Subject Headings (MeSH) list of Index Medicus should be used; if suitable MeSH terms are not available for recently introduced terms, present terms may be used"[3] (see Chapter 1 and Appendix 1).

Introduction

Finally we arrive at the I in IMRAD. The introduction should identify the problem you set out to solve. In general terms, the introduction should cover three areas:

- *Problem statement*: What is the general nature of the problem that merits valuable journal space and the reader's attention?
- *Background and work to date*: What are the most pertinent published studies that relate to the problem?
- *The research question*: What is the specific, focused question that you set out to answer?

The Problem

The introduction classically opens with a broadly stated and virtually unassailable generalization about the problem. In the report of discussing a risk factor for age-related macular degeneration, the authors begin, "Age-related macular degeneration (AMD) is a burden to the elderly population, and its consequences are increasing because treatment options are limited" (Seddon JM, Gensler G, Milton RC, Klein ML, Rifai N. Association between C-reactive protein and age-related macular degermation. JAMA 2004;291(6):704–710).

As the introduction goes on, the authors state, "Many factors associated with AMD are also related to cardiovascular disease." And that brings us, in the next paragraph, to inflammatory biomarkers, such as C-reactive protein.

Background

Describe the key work that has been done on the topic to date. In the words of the uniform requirements, "Give only strictly pertinent references."[3] Do not present an exhaustive literature review dating back to the Renaissance. Be very selective and include only articles that have a direct bearing on your research question.

Research Question
State clearly the question you are trying to answer. One focused question is better than many. The question may be stated as a query or perhaps as a hypothesis, but often is phrased as a statement of intent: In the trial of laboring in water, the research question is stated: "Our current trial therefore compares labour in water with augmentation in nulliparous women with dystocia." The swearing surgeon report states, "We therefore assessed to what extent the use of foul language by surgeons is a myth. We also tried to identify the surgical specialties where swearing is most common."

To inform the reader as to what your study is all about, it is vital that you articulate the research question at the end of the introduction. I wish that writers of research reports would all do so and would frame their research questions as direct queries or even as hypotheses. For example, the authors of the paper on provider continuity and total health care costs state the question right in the title: "Provider continuity in family medicine: does it make a difference in total health care costs?" However, most authors are less explicit, and I have learned to be content with research questions stated as (in the macular degeneration study): "Therefore we examined the relationship between CRP levels and AMD in the multicenter Age-Related Eye Disease Study (AREDS)."

Technical Issues
When writing your introduction, use the present tense when describing the general nature of the problem and the background work. Then the research question, if presented as a statement, is usually in past tense, as in the examples above.

The uniform requirements advise, "Do not include data or conclusions from the work being reported."[3] Not everyone agrees with this stance. Both Day[1] and Whimster[2] advocate stating the conclusions early in the article, and not keeping the reader in suspense, as you would with a whodunit mystery novel. The best spot for the important implication for clinical practice may be in the introduction. In this area where controversy exists, use your best judgment, based on the data you are presenting.

Methods

The Methods section, sometimes called Participants and Methods or perhaps Methods and Materials, should describe a logical experimental approach. Because this section presents a number of topics, subheadings are often used. In the Methods section of the article mentioned above about flu vaccine and ear infections, the authors used the following headings: Participants, Procedures, Vaccine, Surveillance for Otitis Media, Influenza Surveillance, Immunogenicity, Safety Evaluation, Health Care Utilization, and Statistical Analysis. The paper on laboring in water also includes a full spectrum of Methods subheadings: Design, Study Population, Intervention, Sample Size, Randomization and Recruitment, Outcome Measures, and Statistical Analysis.

No Methods subheadings were used for the paper relating provider continuity and total health care costs.

Fundamentally, this section needs to describe the subjects, what you did to them, and what statistical methods you used. After writing the first draft of the Methods section, ask yourself whether what you are presenting allows *reproducibility*. That is, could a trained investigator replicate your study, given the information you have provided?

Methods should not include numerical data, which should be presented in the Results section.

Subjects

Describe the subjects studied, including age, gender, and other important characteristics that may be pertinent to the study. Uniform requirements recommends, when such descriptors are important, that authors "should avoid terms such as 'race,' which lacks precise biological meaning, and use alternative descriptors such as 'ethnicity' or 'ethnic group' instead."[3]

State also whether any potential subjects were excluded and why they were excluded, if there is a meaningful reason. For example, in the study of laboring in water, only nulliparous women were studied; therefore, multiparous women were excluded.

Method

Here you describe what was actually done to the subjects. Be sure to identify all drugs by generic name; adding the trade name is optional, but is useful for the practicing clinician. Be sure to include doses and routes of administration.

Statistics

Describe the statistical methods used, "with enough detail to enable a knowledgeable reader with access to the original data to verify the reported results."[3] This generally means identifying specific tests used. In the study of laboring under water, for instance, the authors report, "We analyzed results on an intention to treat basis. We compared rates of epidural analgesia and operative delivery between groups using Pearson's χ^2 tests and presented results as relative risks with 95% confidence limits."

The uniform requirements recommend that authors "put a general description of (statistical) methods in the Methods section. When data are summarized in the Results section, specify the statistical methods used to analyze them."[3]

Results

What did you discover? Describe your findings in a logical sequence and do so fully, yet succinctly. Stick with the approach that the informed reader should be able to use to replicate the statistical analysis. Provide all data that were analyzed on the way to your conclusions, and show the outcomes of the statistical analysis that you described under Methods.

I have sometimes said, only partly in jest, that the ideal Results section has a single sentence, "The results are presented in Table 1," followed by a carefully constructed table. In reality, presenting research results is never this simple, but the use of tables and figures can help organize numbers in ways that cannot be accomplished in words. Keep in mind that tables and figures are expensive for the journal to produce and are a leading source of error. On balance, however, most Results sections benefit from one or more tables or figures.

Tables and figures for all types of publication model are discussed in detail in Chapter 4. Here I will only emphasize the importance of creating a legend for each that explains the table so that it can be reasonably understood without the accompanying text. That is, a lecturer can incorporate your table with its legend into a PowerPoint presentation (with credit to you, of course).

Tables and figures should not duplicate data presented in the text. Select only one location to present the numbers.

Discussion

In Chapter 1, I stated that each article must face the "So what?" question. The Discussion section must answer that question. The discussion should do so by stating the relationships among facts discovered, relating them to prior studies (the ones you mentioned earlier in the introduction), and postulating what it may all mean—the conclusions. Discuss the results, but do not restate what has already been said under Results.

The Holy Grail in all of this is *generalizability*, a neologism that is not in Microsoft Word's spell checker or *Dorland's Medical Dictionary*, but that all researchers recognize. Does what you have found apply only to your group of subjects, a weakness of the small sample or the single-institution study? Or can the results found be generalized to similar patients elsewhere, the obvious advantage of the large, multicenter trial such as the AREDS macular degeneration study?

State any weaknesses of the study design, or these will surely be described by reviewers or in letters to the editor. The Discussion section is also where you should describe any factors that may have biased collection of the data, such as unexpected events, attrition of subjects, or mid-study changes in methods, such as terminating one of the study groups.

In the last paragraph (where the grazing reader may go right after reading the abstract), present a summary of your conclusions and their implications. Then state the implications for practice, the generalizablity of your work. Write this paragraph very carefully. It represents the outcome of months of work.

References

Your references are where you have obtained information, and indicate your knowledge of prior work in the area of your research. A focused list of citations is more valuable to your reader—and to you, as author—than a very long list of unselected papers.

References serve other purposes. Readers often use them as part of their own research on topics. For these individuals, your list is already a little out of date by the time it is published, but it can be useful at times. Your reference list also represents a sort of "merit badge" for the authors, indicating that you valued their papers enough to cite them as credible sources.

When using a reference citation to support a statement, be sure that you are conveying the actual meaning of the author. I have seen too many references used to support statements when the paper cited says something entirely different.

The technical considerations of presenting references are similar for all publication models, and are presented in Chapter 4. Here I will list just a few additional suggestions and comments:

- Uniform Requirements recommend that you avoid citing abstracts as references.[3]
- If in doubt in listing the name of a journal, write it out, because, for example, "Psych" could mean psychiatry or psychology.
- By custom, a journal with a single word title, such as *Nature* or *Science*, is written in full and is not abbreviated.
- A paper accepted for publication, but not yet published, can be cited as "in press." If the paper is published before your article goes to press, the citation can be updated in page proofs to add the details of publication.
- Because the site of electronic citations can change, the author citing a Web site should print out a copy of the online material, in case it is requested later.
- Never cite a source you have not read and copied for your files.

Acknowledgments

Some papers have a final section listing those who assisted with the work. This includes "all contributors who do not meet the criteria for authorship, such as a person who provided purely technical help, writing assistance, or a department chair who provided only general support."[3] If financial or material support has not been disclosed elsewhere, it should be included here.

There is one important caveat: Be sure that all the people who you thank are pleased to be acknowledged and that they actually agree with the substance of the paper. Being mentioned allows readers to infer that those acknowledged support the data and conclusions. For this reason, you must have written permission from all persons listed in the acknowledgments. Some journals have specific online forms for this purpose; others will accept a signed note on a letterhead.

THOUGHTS ABOUT RESEARCH REPORTS

The section above presents a structured approach to writing what must be a structured article. What follows are some random thoughts about writing a research report.

Quality Writing and Research Design

Medical composition is a laudable skill, one that we should all work to improve. When it comes to writing a report of a clinical research study, however, medical writing skill must take a back seat to research design. Have you ever read a research report and wondered whether the skillful prose— perhaps composed chiefly by an editorial assistant—masks spurious methods or unjustified conclusions? As Dirckx[7] has written, one should guard "against the temptation to cover his lack of information with a rhetorical snow job, to palm off muddy thinking under a veneer of smooth writing."

Stating What You Really Think

Reports of clinical research studies are often written by committee; the members seek consensus on what will appear in print. Perhaps this is why the final version of the paper does not always reflect the opinions of some researchers on the team and often does not reflect the diversity of author opinions. Richard Horton, editor of *The Lancet*, surveyed contributors to 10 research articles published in *The Lancet*. Thirty-six of 54 contributors to the 10 articles responded to questions in a qualitative analysis. The research question was: "To determine whether the views expressed in a research paper are accurate representations of contributors' opinions about the research being reported."[8] The study found unreported concerns about study weaknesses, and disagreements among authors about findings and their significance. The study concludes that one remedy for the problem of suppressed opinions may be structured Discussion sections in research papers, as we now see in Abstracts.

Writing and Research Mentors

A mentor can be a big help in medical writing. Without question, my most influential mentor was the late Charles Visokay, M.D., medical editor at Harper and Row Medical Publishers and subsequently with Springer-Verlag–New York publishers. Chuck guided me through publication of three authored medical reference books and then gave me the opportunity to edit a new major reference book at a time in my life when I was a solo country doctor.

As much as having a writing mentor can help, it is not a necessity. Research is different. Research is best undertaken in teams. Members of the team bring different skills, and the group effort allows individuals to maintain commitment. Mentors can be especially important team members, who provide nurturing and guidance. They help keep young researchers on track. Hoff[9] writes: "When I finished medical school, I did not intend to do research as part of my life in surgery. That all changed when I met a mentor who inspired me during my training days. I had some protected time, assembled space and equipment, developed a hypothesis, and went to it. I'll never forget my first experiment and publication. Frankly, it was my best."

Research Reports and Your Academic Career

Earlier in the chapter I mentioned that research reports are very important in academic advancement. Let me tell you just how important they are.

When one is a candidate for academic promotion—let's say from assistant to associate professor—a dossier is assembled to support the promotion. This task falls to the faculty member working, I hope, with an experienced mentor or guide. The packet often has several hundred pages of documents, the most important of which may be the publications list.

The currency in academic medicine is the *creation of new knowledge*. This means research studies, with reports published in research journals. Each faculty member's dossier is evaluated by the institution's Promotion and Tenure (P&T) Committee, which includes a number of basic science researchers and perhaps some professors from schools other than medicine or nursing. These individuals very carefully review the publication list, which must pass muster. The P&T committee evaluates each promotion candidate against his or her position description, and research faculty are held to the highest standards of publication. Even "clinical" faculty members, often with patient loads much like colleagues in private practice, and nonphysician educator faculty must produce written evidence of creating new knowledge if they are to be promoted.

A publication list with only review articles and literature reviews is not enough. The members of the P&T committee, especially the nonclinician basic scientists, will be looking at the number and quality of research reports. They will also look at where the reports were published. Was your seminal paper published in the *Mid-Valley Regional Medical Journal* or in the *Annals of Internal Medicine*?

All of this is to say that, if you are a clinician in academic medicine, your career advancement depends on publishing reports of original research. Writing review articles, book reviews, and letters to the editor allows you to get early writing experience and entries on your curriculum vitae. In the end, you will need to conduct and report clinical or educational research.

Getting Your Research Report in Print

General Douglas MacArthur once said, "There is no substitute for victory." In academic medicine, there is no substitute for publication. You can have a brilliant idea, perform groundbreaking research, and write the results with great proficiency, but if the paper is not published—so that it can be cited, criticized, or praised—then the effort has been largely wasted. The advancement of science depends on sharing of knowledge in print. Chapter 10 discusses how to achieve publication, for your research report or other publication models.

REFERENCES

1. Day RA. How to write and publish a scientific paper. Westport, CT: Oryx, 1998;12, 34.
2. Whimster WF. Biomedical research: how to plan, publish and present it. New York: Springer-Verlag, 1997;101, 105.
3. International Committee of Medical Journal Editors. Uniform requirements for manuscripts submitted to biomedical journals. Updated October 2001. www.icmje.org.
4. Strasburger VC. Righting medical writing. JAMA 1985;254(13): 1789–1790.
5. Rennie D, Glass RM. Structuring abstracts to make them more informative. JAMA 1991;266(1):116–117.
6. Journal of the American Medical Association. Instructions for authors. Available at: http://jama.ama-assn.org/ifora_current/dtl.
7. Dirckx J. Dx+Rx: a physician's guide to medical writing. Boston: G.K. Hall; 1977:99.
8. Horton R. The hidden research paper. JAMA 2002;287: 2775–2778.
9. Hoff JT. Research by academic surgeons. Am J Surg 2003; 185(1):13–15.

10

Getting Your Writing Published

You have had a great idea for a review article, case report, editorial, or letter to the editor. Maybe you did a clinical research project. You developed the concept—how you would handle the idea. You have written the paper, revised it at least three times (see Chapter 3), and had it critiqued by your harshest reviewer colleague before preparing the final draft. In short, you have been able to write it up. These are all important steps; the next is getting your work in print. Notice that I say, "Next step," which I will explain at the end of the chapter.

What follows are hints as to how to get your work published. The advice is general, and applies to all the publication models discussed in the book, not only to research reports.

Fundamentally, publication follows an invitation by an editor that is accepted by the author. Of course, there will be peer review, editing changes, and sometimes a major revision. But, following negotiated changes, author and editor must both say, "Yes." And it is a good idea to achieve the consensual affirmative as soon as possible, because the material in a medical article is going out of date as the ink dries on the manuscript page.

In fact, you and the journal editor have consistent goals. You, as author, want your work in print as soon as possible. The editor needs high-quality articles for publication, in most cases each month. You and the editor need one another. As King[1] writes, "Authors and publishers thus live in symbiosis. The unpublished manuscript accomplishes nothing for its author, and a journal without manuscripts speedily dies."

PLANNING YOUR ARTICLE SUBMISSION

Submitting Your Article to the Right Journal

Planning the journal for first submission is an important step that should begin as you conceptualize the paper, as discussed in Chapter 1. In many cases, you will call or send an e-mail query to the editor to see whether there is some interest in the topic. This publication then becomes your "target journal."

Pay attention to how often the journal publishes papers in your topic area. What topics are generally presented in the journal? If you have a paper on a general medical topic, such as irritable bowel syndrome, depression, or chest pain, your range of possibilities is wide. If your paper describes a urologic surgical procedure or a method of teaching psychologic assessment of the geriatric patient, your choices are much more limited.

Sometimes you will sense an unmet need. If your research shows that the *Annals of Internal Medicine* has published no articles on gynecologic topics over the past few years, that finding can mean one of two things: either the journal editor considers gynecologic articles outside the scope of the journal, or the editor is eagerly awaiting a submission in this area, and will welcome your paper on current therapy of vaginitis.

In selecting your target journal, consider the following factors:

The Variety of Article Formats

Some journals accept almost no articles that are not research reports. Others limit themselves to review articles. Some publish case reports; other journals never do so. In some journals you will find invited editorials—that is, written by persons who are not the editor of the journal. In other journals, only the editor writes the editorials. Here are two ways to check on the variety of article formats published: review several recent issues of the journal, which is also helpful in determining the scope of topics, the writing style, and what authors are publishing in the journal; review the instructions for authors, which will probably describe the types of article published, with some guidelines for the preparation of each.

The Journal's Impact Factor

For the author submitting a research report, the impact factor becomes a two-edged sword. On one hand, the impact factor of the journal has been found to be "more important than any other variable, suggesting that the journal in which a study is published may be as important as traditional measures of study quality in ensuring dissemination."[2] This means that study methods and design did not predict the frequency of citations for a study or the prestige of the citing journals. Simply stated, the key factor in having your work widely cited is the journal in which it is published. For a fuller discussion of the journal impact factor and how it is determined, go to Chapter 5.

On the other hand, and this is why I bring up the impact factor again, a journal's high impact factor can reduce your chances of acceptance. Every writer knows about the importance of where one's work is published, even if few know how to calculate the impact factor. The most prestigious journals receive huge numbers of submissions. The most submissions of all are likely to go the major broad-based journals, with acceptance rates often below 10%.

Aiming High: The Controversy

Some investigators submit their papers first to one of the most prestigious journals. Of course there is a slim chance of acceptance, but the authors know this is very unlikely. What they seek is a critical review of the paper by experts. In recommending rejection, the peer reviewers will identify the weaknesses of the paper. This allows the author to fix the problems before submitting the paper to what was always the target journal.

One disadvantage to such a practice is that it delays publication. The turnaround time in peer review and editorial decision making is measured in months. For a paper that has very timely data, this delay may actually work against publication.

The larger question is the ethical issue of seeking what is really a free consultation on your paper, when you know that your chances of acceptance approach zero. Yet one goal of volunteer peer reviewers must be to help investigators and authors prepare the best papers possible.

Working with Journal Editors

Working with editors means recognizing and respecting what they want from you. Norton,[3] an assistant editor of the

Journal of the American Academy of Dermatology, writes, "I would be proud if every article published in the Journal were novel, interesting and important—in other words, if every article were both readable and worth reading. (I'd also like it if every article were eloquent, funny, and short.) The Editors would love to receive manuscripts that are perfect when first submitted, but these papers probably don't exist. The peer review system is intended to select the most worthwhile papers and nudge them along toward that elusive perfection."

"Read the instructions, Grandpa." This is my 5-year-old granddaughter's directive when mixing ingredients to make pancakes, starting a board game, or trying to operate a new electronic gadget. My granddaughter is on the right track. Journal editors earnestly wish that more authors would actually read—and follow—the instructions for authors. Failure to do so results in extra work for both editor and author. It can cause delays, as the manuscript is returned for the missing pieces. Sometimes failure to follow directions can result in summary rejection (see below), simply because it was egregiously nonconforming.

Good Manuscripts and Bad: What Editors Think

Here is what one editor thinks about good and bad articles:

> Wonderful articles are alike in so many ways. They have a concise introduction that proposes a testable hypothesis, a methods section with a good study design, a results section in which the statistical analysis addresses clinical relevance as well as statistical significance, and a discussion in which points are made succinctly and are based on evidence, not conjecture. In wonderful articles, the prose is clear, fluent, and direct. On the other hand, unhappy articles are often uniquely bad, each with its particular combination of distinctive flaws.[3]

In an insightful, but humorous editorial in JAMA, Grouse[4] identifies a "rogue's gallery of medical manuscripts." The following describes a few of the perpetrators.

The Clone

The clone is born as a researcher attempts to publish two or more papers based on data in a single study. The act of submitting clone articles is sometimes called fractionated publication, salami science, or duplicate publication. Von Elm et al[5] reviewed 56 systematic literature reviews that included 1131 main articles. They report, "Sixty articles were published twice, 13 three times, 3 four times, and 2 five times."

Academic institutions must bear some responsibility for this behavior, as educators carefully count the number of publications at promotion time. Journals contribute to the problem with a reluctance to publish long research reports. Nevertheless, the clone uses valuable journal space in presenting background material, methodology and often-similar conclusions in several papers.

The Chain Letter

The chain letter is a variation on the clone. In a chain letter, a research group lets each member be first author by submitting an ongoing series of papers that present just a little more data from an ongoing study plus a great deal of previously published results. Each version of the chain letter varies in the list of authors and in the title of the article.

The Attention Grabber

In this manuscript the authors may have conducted perfectly good research, but they postulate conclusions that go beyond their data. In many cases, the discussion offers hope in the diagnosis or treatment of disease that is sure to be reported in the media. The worst case is when the authors release their findings to the media just as their scientific article goes to press.

The Shell Game

Simply stated, a shell game occurs when an author submits the identical paper to more than one journal at a time. Playing the shell game is risky and some say unethical. The player "wins" when one journal accepts the paper, and it is rejected by all the others. The player loses when two or more journals accept the article, and all but one must be told (or learn) of the ruse. The shell game wastes editors' time. It can make for duplicate publication if the author doesn't withdraw the paper from all but one publication. Journal editors hate shell game players.

The Sneak Attack

In his paper, the author launches a missile aimed at a colleague in the field. The Background or Discussion section of the paper contains a cleverly crafted criticism of the colleague's work, perhaps including an attack on the individual.

The Zombie

This describes a manuscript that never dies. When a journal rejects an article in no uncertain terms, it means that the editor does not want to see the manuscript again. The author's job is to make any needed changes, and then submit the article elsewhere. Do not let your manuscript become a zombie by resubmitting it without an invitation to do so.

TECHNICAL REQUIREMENTS FOR PUBLICATION

By now you have selected the best journal for first submission, contacted the editor or decided why you should not do so, and made sure your manuscript will not end up in the "rogue's gallery." It is time to take care of the last technical details of manuscript submission.

Submission Letter

The first item in your packet will be a submission letter, which should accompany every manuscript from research report to letter to the editor. Also sometimes called the "cover letter," the submission letter provides information about your paper and about you as the author. The letter should be addressed to the journal editor, by name. Identify the title of the paper just before the salutation in the letter. Table 10.1 describes the contents of a comprehensive submission letter.

TABLE 10.1. Contents of cover letter accompanying an article manuscript submitted to a medical journal

Letter item	What to include
Introductory paragraph	Identify the accompanying manuscript and indicate that you are submitting it to be considered for publication. In some instances, you should identify the type of paper you are submitting, e.g., report of original research, brief report, case report, or other format.
Word count	Cite the number of words in the manuscript. Your word processing program will give you the needed number.
Specific author contributions	Many journals ask that you describe each author's specific contribution to the research and writing. For example, did an author recruit the subjects, collect data, provide statistical analysis, or edit the manuscript?
Contact author	Identify the one author who will respond to correspondence and who can answer questions about the study. Provide full contact information.
Copyright relinquishment	Most journals insist that the cover letter relinquish copyright if the article is published. See the journal's instructions to authors to determine if this is needed in the letter and, if so, to note the exact wording to be used.
Conflict of interest disclosure	Describe any industry sponsorship of the study, contractural agreements with industry, consulting or speaking agreements, or even stock ownership if there might be a perceived conflict of interest.
Author approval	State that the manuscript has been read and approved by all the authors, that the requirements for authorship have been met, and that each author believes that the manuscript represents honest work.[6]
Duplicate submission or publication	State that the contents of the paper have not been published previously and that the manuscript has not been submitted elsewhere. State if an abstract has been presented at a scientific meeting.
Special requests	Try to avoid special requests. However, in the case of cutting-edge scientific research, there may be a valid reason for requesting that a certain individual not be used as a peer reviewer.
Thank you	Thank the editor for considering your manuscript for publication.
Signatures	All authors should sign the submission letter.
Enclosures	Be sure to send the requested number of manuscript copies, and also any required compact disk or other materials. Consider sending a copy of your one-page, abbreviated curriculum vitae.

Title Page

The title page gives important data about the paper and the authors. The title page should include the following items, which are consistent with the recommendations of the International Committee of Medical Journal Editors[6] and the instructions for submission to the *New England Journal of Medicine*:[7]

- The article's title: be descriptive but concise
- Each author's name, academic degree(s), and institutional affiliation
- The name of the department(s) and institution(s) where the work was done
- Disclaimers, if any are appropriate
- The corresponding author's name and full contact information
- The name and address of the person to whom reprint requests should be addressed, or a statement that no reprints will be available
- Sources of support, such as grants
- A running head (a short version of the title) that will appear on each manuscript page

Literature Review Update

Just before submitting the manuscript, repeat your literature review. Important papers may have touched on your topic since you did your original literature search. Be sure that there has been no "breakthrough" study that should be included in your article. Assure yourself also that no one has recently published a paper just like yours. Having someone beat you to publication on a topic should not discourage you from submitting, but you should know that the game has changed.

What to Submit and in What Order

When you finally have collected all the pieces, it is time to assemble your submission packet. Unless specifically instructed otherwise, assemble your packet of materials as follows:

- Submission letter
- Title page
- Abstract
- Key words
- Body of the text
- Acknowledgments
- References
- Tables with legends, each on a separate page
- Figures with legends, each on a separate page

If requested, include a computer diskette or compact disk.

The journal will almost certainly request an original and several copies of manuscripts. Check the instructions to authors if you are submitting artwork. Will it be acceptable to submit one original and several copies of a figure, or will you need multiple copies of original art or photographs?

When you are all ready to place your work in an envelope, review the checklist in Table 10.2 to help assure that you are not forgetting anything.

TABLE 10.2. Manuscript checklist for journal article or book chapter submission

_____ Double-space the entire manuscript, including references.
_____ Use 12-point font unless the instructions specify otherwise.
_____ Leave the right margin of the manuscript unjustified (i.e., ragged).
_____ Identify all abbreviations when first used in the text.
_____ Use nonproprietary names of drugs.
_____ Check all references for accuracy and completeness.
_____ Confirm that all references are cited in the text.
_____ Be sure you have disclosed any possible conflict of interest.
_____ For all borrowed materials, send a consent form signed by the copyright holder.
_____ Include informed consent to use images that may identify human subjects.
_____ Submit the requested number of copies of the manuscript, tables, and figures.
_____ If submitting by e-mail, include text, tables, and figures in a single file, if possible.
_____ Keep a copy of everything, which will be used later to check proofs.

Packing and Mailing Tips

Pack your manuscript as you would a family heirloom. You have put a lot of work into the article. Don't risk a problem at this stage. More manuscripts than you might imagine are damaged, delayed, or lost in the mail.

Do not staple anything related to the manuscript. The publisher may want to make photocopies for files, and staples jam photocopiers. Also, be careful with paper clips, which can damage artwork and photographs. If you must use paper clips, use large ones that cause less damage. Never write on the back of a photograph; identify the figure by writing on an adhesive label, and then apply the label to the back of the photo.

Computer diskettes and compact disks should be sent in special padded containers or between sheets of heavy cardboard.

All artwork should be 8½ by 11 inches in size or smaller, unless you have a special agreement with the editor. Large artwork is difficult to ship and to handle in the office.

I like to enclose a self-addressed, stamped postcard for the editorial staff member to return to me, letting me know that my package has arrived.

Finally, be sure to keep a paper copy of your entire manuscript, even if everything is on your hard drive. I know an author whose manuscript was only on his computer; he had no paper copy. You can guess the rest of the story. Luckily, the submitted manuscript was returned after review, and he was able to scan everything to his computer. Then he kept a printed copy.

Some Mistakes Made in Submitting Manuscripts

The discussion above will help you avoid most manuscript submission errors. Here are some additional topics.

Relying on Your Spell Checker

Your Microsoft Word spelling and grammar utility is excellent, but it will not detect all errors. For example, type in the following:

> Eye no hat correct spelling is important, and sew I was care full to us the spell checker.

My Microsoft spell checker accepted this sentence as correct.

Touting Your Paper

Do not use your submission letter to tell the editor that yours is a very important paper. Editors look at many papers, and can recognize those that are important, especially with the advice of peer reviewers. Your paper is not a used car to be "sold," claiming to report the greatest advance since Wilhelm Conrad Röntgen took a snapshot of his wife's hand in 1895.

Seeking Perfection

Earlier in this chapter, I quoted Norton about the quest for "elusive perfection." In fact, your paper will never be perfect, either as to content or manuscript preparation. In writing fact, conclusions, and opinion, do not undertake multiple, but trivial, revisions. At some time you must say, as all writers and artists must eventually do, that this is as good as I can reasonably make it, and I am going to declare it done.

As to making the manuscript perfect, let me quote from the instructions to authors of the journal *Academic Medicine*:[8] "The editors will make reasonable allowance for minor deviations from these technical specifications so long as they do not interfere with reading, reviewing, or editing the manuscript. Major deviations, however, may lead the editors to require corrections before the manuscript is processed." The point is that you should do your very best when writing a paper. However, do not fret about whether the terminal page numbers in references should be written in full or abbreviated. Such "minor deviations" will not cause rejection, and perseveration over trivia can only interfere with your writing success.

THE REVIEW PROCESS

Your paper has been received by the journal and has been sent for review. Your article was not summarily rejected, sent back immediately by the editor as being "not appropriate for consideration by the journal." That would have meant that the editor believed the work to be outside the journal's field or that it is libelous, blasphemous, or totally irrational.[9] You have passed the first hurdle. Things are now in the hands of the peer reviewers.

Peer Review

The Role and Duties of the Peer Reviewer

The journal editor considers the peer reviewers who will review your paper to be familiar with your topic. Many are senior academicians and investigators. All are volunteers, and they do a lot of work for no pay. Peer reviewers, sometimes called referees, can be a very big help to you, even if your paper is ultimately rejected.

How are peer reviewers chosen? Each journal has a panel of peer reviewers who have been recruited by the editor. If you wish to be a peer reviewer, send a letter and your curriculum vitae to the journal editor and volunteer to serve. State the areas in which you have some expertise and are willing to review papers. The editor will reply, and perhaps add you to the review team. Editors want their peer reviewers to have certain traits. Peer reviewers should be knowledgeable in the topic under consideration, intellectually honest, and time-sensitive. The author and editor cannot wait 3 months for a paper to be reviewed. In reviewing reports of clinical studies, a peer reviewer should know research methodology and basic statistical analysis. In the end, the peer reviewer helps to improve the paper, making it clearer, more informative, and often shorter—even if the paper is ultimately rejected by the journal. (Remember that the paper will then be revised and submitted to the next journal on the list.) These are exactly the traits you hope for in the reviewer who evaluates your paper.

The duties of a peer reviewer can be summarized as follows:

- Accept a paper to review only if the job can be completed promptly.
- Agree to referee papers only in areas of the reviewer's expertise.
- Maintain confidentiality about the paper.
- Disclose any possible conflict of interest, and decline a review if there is any potential difficulty.
- Write a thoughtful review that is honest and free of bias.

■ Aim to make the paper the best it can be, balancing criticism with suggestions for improvement.

■ Avoid excessively harsh comments, especially those that could be interpreted as a personal attack on the author(s).

The peer reviewer never contacts the author directly. In most cases, but not all, the name of the author is not present on the paper being reviewed. Remember that above I stated that the author's name goes only on the title page, which is not sent to the peer reviewer. There are exceptions. The last paper I reviewed contained the names of the authors and there had been no effort to "blind" the review. Even when the names of authors and institutions are absent in blinded reviews, the peer reviewer who is working actively in the field can often tell the source of the paper based on the topic, methods, and even writing style.

I think of the roles of a peer reviewer and a practicing clinician as similar. Both are expected to exhibit ethical behavior and to be committed to providing high-quality service. Both the reviewer and clinician should be knowledgeable, capable, and thorough in what they do. Both have the ability to examine details while keeping a broad perspective. Both are reliable and trustworthy, and believe that they serve a worthy purpose.

The Role and Duties of the Editor
The editor makes the final decision about acceptance or rejection of an article. Of course, an editor's decision is based strongly on the recommendations of the peer reviewers. Although it is significant that most papers seem to go to three reviewers, not two or four, the final decision is not a "vote." Editors are paid to make judgments, and they do so.

Editors, like peer reviewers, must be honest, ethical, unbiased, responsible, and detail-oriented. They must also be literate, knowledgeable, and compulsive as to deadlines. After all, most journals must be published every month, some more often.

The editor serves as the buffer between the author and the peer reviewers. As such the editor must be able to deal with authors who are disappointed or angry. In other cases, the problem is tardy or careless authors. A good editor can handle all these problems with tact and grace.

What Actually Happens

Here is a quick summary of what occurs when you submit a paper. Your article is logged in the system and probably given an identification number. You should be sent a notification that your package has been received.

Next the editor or assistant editor reviews the article quickly to see whether it merits peer review. As discussed above, articles with topics outside the journal's scope or those that are carelessly prepared will be immediately rejected and returned to the author.

Those that survive the initial screen are sent to referees for peer review. Each referee prepares an evaluation. Most evaluations have two parts; one part is for the editor's eyes only, and one part is sent to you, the author. The part sent to you can be quite valuable or not, as discussed below.

When all reviews are received, the editor makes a decision and lets you know the outcome of the process. If you have not heard about a decision in a reasonable time, let's say 8 weeks from the time of submission, it is a good idea to contact the journal. For example, your paper may be collecting dust while the assistant awaits receipt of a third review, due from a referee who has left for a 4-month trek in Nepal. Some journals offer a way to keep track of the process. For example, the NEJM provides PaperTRAIL as a Web site to allow "an author to obtain a rapid, confidential update on his or her manuscript."[10]

Possible Responses from the Journal Editor

The journal editor's decision will come as a letter that indicates one the following: rejection, revision, or acceptance.

Rejection Letter

Was it a coincidence that, on the evening before I sat down to write this section of the chapter, our local newspaper carried a Peanuts cartoon about rejection? (*The Oregonian*, March 5,

2004). Snoopy opened the mailbox to find a letter that said, "Dear Contributor. We are returning your dumb story. Note that we have not included our return address. We have moved to a new office, and we don't want you to know where we are."

The rejection letter is the one you really don't want to receive. The editor will probably avoid the word "reject," and instead will euphemistically characterize your paper as "unacceptable" or state that it "does not meet the journal's needs." Basically the editor is saying that, after careful review, your paper will not be published in their journal. Furthermore, he or she believes that it cannot be revised or improved to make it publishable. The editor does not want to see your paper again.

Unless you have had the bad luck to compete with an article in press that is very similar to yours, the rejection will be attributed chiefly to the evaluations of the referees. These comments will usually be sent to you, and you should read them very carefully. The decision to reject will be based on one or more of the reasons listed in Table 10.3.

Your first reaction will be denial. Could this editor really have rejected my paper? Could there be a mistake? Maybe this rejection slip was meant for someone else. Then you read the reviewer comments and become annoyed, actually furious. How could they miss the point of my paper? Did the referees read the paper at all?

Next you settle down and consider appealing the decision. Should you request reconsideration? Actually, this sometimes

TABLE 10.3. Classic causes of article rejection

Unimportant topic
Outdated information
Inadequate literature review
Faulty scientific method
Conclusions that are inconsistent with the data
Poor structure to the article
Poor writing
Suspected bias, plagiarism, duplicate publication, inappropriate criticism of colleagues and their work, or other ethical concerns

works. Whimster[9] estimates success "in perhaps 15% of cases." Your appeal must be rational and civilized. Describing the referees as troglodytes will not help you. A reasonable appeal letter should politely refute the reviewers' criticisms point by point, citing evidence. Show how your paper will be especially important to the journal's readers and how this point may have been overlooked. Indicate any recent publications that validate your findings and conclusions. Type your brief, let it sit for a day or two to cool off, and then revise to expunge any hint of anger. Then mail the appeal letter, and prepare to be rejected again.

Then sadness sets in. Maybe I am not cut out to be a medical writer. Perhaps I should spend my spare time working in the yard or playing golf. How could I have ever had the hubris to think that I could get my work in print?

By this time have you recognized the classical stages of bereavement—denial, anger, bargaining, depression, and acceptance—described by Elisabeth Kübler-Ross?[11]

The final step is to accept the judgment of journal number one. At this point, you should study the comments of the reviewers and use this opportunity to improve the paper. Seek the nuggets of truth in the reviewers' remarks. Yes, I know that at least one of the reviewers seems to have totally misunderstood the paper, and maybe there is a message there. Make the appropriate revisions and use this time to update the literature search and references, especially if a few months have passed. Then submit the paper to another journal. Do this soon to help prevent becoming discouraged. As a hint, subsequent submissions are sometimes more successful when sent to more specialized journals.

When sending the paper to another journal, be sure to send a new clean copy. The manuscript returned by the rejecting journal may have pencil marks, staple holes, or coffee stains. When preparing the second submission, read the journal's instructions and make sure your manuscript complies with its technical requirements, which are sure to differ from those of the previous journal. Basically, the second submission should have no indication that this is not the first time the paper has left your desk.

Submitting a clean manuscript is professional, and is courteous to the editor of journal number two. There is, of course, the chance that one of the reviewers for the second journal may be the same person who was a referee for the first publication, an occurrence most likely in limited scientific fields.

I recommend that you save all rejection letters. Put them in a folder in the back of your file. Medical writers all receive many rejection letters, and the file may eventually overflow. Years from now you will read them and chuckle.

Revision Letter

This is a much better letter to receive than the rejection letter. Be aware that the revision letter, sometimes called the modification letter, can be misleading. It can begin with the cunning phrase, "I regret to inform you that your paper does not meet requirements in its present form." Oh, sadness and gloom! But read on. The next sentence may be, "However, if you make revisions as suggested by the peer reviewers, we will be pleased to reconsider your submission." Hooray! This is actually a conditional acceptance letter. If you agree with the suggestions offered by the referees, make the recommended changes and thank the reviewers in your "resubmission letter." Your resubmission letter should also indicate where changes were made and how they relate to the comments of the referees and editor.

In modifying your paper, make only the suggested changes. Do not add new data or conclusions, which can only give the editor and referees something new to criticize. Make surgical repairs and resubmit before the editor has a change of mind.

One dilemma you may face is the "revision letter" that invites you to cut your paper to 500 words for a brief report or shorten to a letter to the editor (see Chapter 7). This calls for some soul-searching, discussion with coauthors, and perhaps consultation with a trusted senior advisor. On one hand, there is virtually certain publication in a journal high on your list. On the other hand, you have to give up on full presentation of your data and conclusions. I can only recommend that your writing team struggle to a unanimous decision.

Acceptance Letter

Someday you might receive the following letter:

> Dear Contributor:
>
> The three referees and I have all read your paper.
> We agree that your methods are brilliant, your results are clearly stated, and the conclusions are logical and important. We have no suggestions to make and wish to publish the paper as submitted.
> Yours truly,
>
> The Editor

But I don't think that letter will ever come. If you submit an article to a major refereed clinical journal and it is accepted upon first submission without a single revision, let me know and I will take you to dinner the next time you are in Portland, Oregon.

Most acceptance letters follow one or more revisions. This is probably a good idea, because the revisions, based on reviewer comments, usually result in better papers in print.

Whose Papers Are Published and Why?

In the next few paragraphs, I share some of the dark secrets of medical publication, especially in regard to research reports. Tell no one what you read next!

About Peer Review

Peer review may not be the pristine process we imagine. Conflicts of interest are rampant, especially in focused research communities. There are only so many investigators who are experts on, as a fanciful example, the new vaccine against male-pattern baldness. Few people would have the expertise to review papers in this area, and all may be at different stages along the same path to a very lucrative discovery. Is it possible that the reviewer might make use of the information in the paper being reviewed? Such use would be unethical, but I am sure that it might happen.

Occasionally review decisions lack the integrity and quality we authors hope for. Strasburger[12] describes the peer-review system in medical journals: "There, one's peers may have a decided self-interest in not seeing a particular article published, may simply not know very much about the subject, or may be inexperienced writers themselves. Reports may be criticized by someone who is an 'inferior,' rather than a 'peer.'"

Your Native Language Matters

If you speak English as your native language, you have an advantage over others around the world. A study by Coates et al[13] found, "The acceptance rate of non-mother English tongue authors is generally a lot lower than that for native English tongue authors." The fundamental issue seems to concern language errors in manuscripts, rather than discrimination against international contributors. Consider yourself, as one who speaks English daily and other languages infrequently or not at all, being required to submit your scientific paper in Russian or Japanese languages. My manuscript would surely be full of grammatical errors. This helps explain the study findings that, in submissions to the journal *Cardiovascular Research*, "The US/UK acceptance rate of 30.4% was higher than for all other countries. The lowest acceptance rate of 9% (Italian) also had the highest error rate."[13] Simply stated, the authors conclude that with articles of equal scientific merit, a poorly written article is more likely to be rejected.

About Authors and Affiliations

One of my all-time favorite articles was published in 1982 in *Behavioral and Brain Sciences*. Authors Peters and Ceci[14] wondered about the adequacy and fairness of peer-review practices. Here is what they did: The authors selected 12 articles by researchers in highly respected United States psychology departments. Each of these articles had been published in a different, prestigious American psychology journal with high rejection rates (80%) and nonblinded peer reviewers. The authors substituted fictitious names and institutions (such as the Tri-Valley Center for Human Potential) for the original. The manuscripts, with only author names and institutions changed, were then formally resubmitted to the same journals that had peer reviewed and published them 18 to 32 months earlier.

What happened to the 12 papers? Thirty-eight editors and reviewers evaluated the altered articles; only three detected the ruse. Nine of the 12 articles were studiously reviewed, resulting in an editorial decision. In the end, eight of the nine were rejected. Sixteen of 18 referees had recommended against publication. In many cases, the referees described "serious methodological flaws."

The authors ponder the possibility "that systematic bias was operating to produce the discrepant reviews. The most obvious candidates as sources of bias in this case would be the authors' status and institutional affiliation."[14]

In getting published, who you are, where you work, what language you speak daily, and who reviews your paper may profoundly influence whether your paper is accepted or rejected.

AFTER YOUR ARTICLE IS ACCEPTED

Finally, the acceptance letter arrives. No more worrying, and no more revisions. Your article is on its way into print. There are now three items to consider: proofreading, preventing errors, and what to do after publication.

Proofreading

Upon acceptance of your article, a copyeditor will mark it up for publication and correct errors of grammar and syntax. The copyeditor is your friend. With a degree in English literature, the copyeditor is there to help you and the editor publish the best article possible. There may be minor alterations to improve clarity and eliminate ambiguity. You may find very long sentences divided into two, and even some subheadings added in long expanses of text. The changes made will reflect standing orders from the editor about style, and should not affect meaning. You may or may not be sent the marked-up manuscript to review. If you are sent the manuscript, ignore marks you do not understand; these are there as directions for the typesetter. There will probably be questions to you as author (Au:). Answer these questions succinctly, and return the manuscript promptly. The journal probably has already reserved space in an upcoming edition.

Although you may or may not see the marked-up manuscript, you will definitely receive proofs to review. Occasionally you will be sent *galley proofs*—your manuscript set in type but not yet formatted to the journal page. Some journals always send galley proofs, while others send galleys only when they anticipate that the author will want to make some more changes.

Read every word in the proofs, making corrections in pencil—not ink. Begin by checking the page proofs against the manuscript. Has anything been omitted or jumbled? This happens. Do all the reference citations appear in the text, and do the numbers match the reference list? Pay special attention to tables and figures. If there are numbers and totals in the paper, get out your calculator to recheck math.

Prior to publication, you will receive page proofs, with your article set in type and formatted to the journal page, perhaps even with the page numbers in place. Here also there may be queries to "Au." You must answer these questions precisely. Do not waffle or give both sides to an answer. The editor is asking you for a decision about an issue in your paper. Make the decision and state what it is.

Keep in mind that proofreading is intended to correct errors. You may be tempted to add new material during proofreading. A new study was published since your paper was submitted, or a new drug has been introduced. If you propose to add to the paper, I advise that you call the editorial office and discuss what you have in mind. Some editors will approve adding sentence or two, or perhaps a reference.

If adding a reference, ask about numbering. In many journals, the author need not renumber all 90 references when adding the 91st in proofs. Instead, go to the appropriate location in the text and in the reference list and add the new number with an "a." Thus, if the new reference follows reference 45, the new addition will be reference 45a as a text citation and also in the reference list. This convenience saves time and cost, and avoids many typesetting errors.

There are proofreader's marks used as shorthand to identify corrections and changes in proofs. These are found in Appendix 2.

Keep a copy of the corrected proofs. You spent valuable time and mental energy on the changes. Assume that the packet you are returning to the journal will get lost in the mail.

Good writing is hard; good proofreading is even harder. Perhaps this is because it is not creative. Proofreading can be mind-numbingly dull, and this is a danger, because it is very easy to have errors escape into print.

About Errors

Whenever I have published a book and have the first copy in my hand, I can unfailingly open the book to the exact page with a misspelled word. It may be the only one in a 1200-page book, but it seems to jump out at me. I am afraid the same will occur with this book.

The University of New South Wales has advertised for a mathematics research assistant who would work in a "3/4 research and 1/3 teaching position." Sometimes mistakes in print are called *errata*, as though the Latin word makes them seem less serious. Errors find their way into print in many ways. Some begin with the author and some with copyediting, but I believe that most occur in typesetting. It really doesn't matter how they occur, it is the author's job to find and eliminate them with careful proofreading.

A paper on eating disorders is titled "Detection, Evaluation, and Treatment of Eating Disorders: The Role of the Primary Care Physician" (Walsh JME, Wheat ME, Freund K. J Gen Intern Med 2000;15(8):577–583). In the conclusion, the authors state: "Primary care *providers* (italics mine) have an important role in detecting and managing eating disorders." Whoops. Somehow between the title and conclusion the authors moved from primary care physicians to primary care providers, the latter being a much larger and diverse group.

If you think errors won't occur, examine Figure 10.1A and B carefully. They are from an article about medical publication. Do you see the error? Hint: The lines in Fig. 10.1B are correctly labeled. Now look at the two arrows pointing to the single line and the other "arrow-less" line in Fig. 10.1A.

One hundred years ago, *The Lancet* apologized for using the words "a sour correspondent," insisting that it should have

(a)

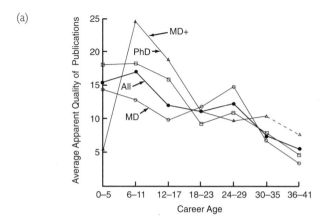

Figure 10.1A

Average apparent quality of publications versus career age for the four-year sample

(b)

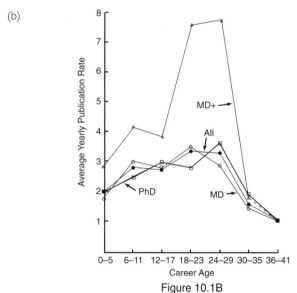

Figure 10.1B

Average yearly publication rate versus career age for faculty in the four-year sample.
The last point on the MD+ curve, career age 36 to 41 years, represents only two faculty
members; therefore, the corresponding portion of the curve has been dotted.

FIGURE 10.1A, B. Figure A has an error in labeling. Figure B is correctly labeled. Can you spot the error in Figure A? (The original captions were: Fig. A, Average apparent quality of publications versus career age for the four-year sample. Fig. B, Average yearly publication rate versus career age for the four-year sample. From: Krumland RB, Gorry GA. Scientific publications of a medical school faculty. J Med Educ 1979;54:876–884. Used with permission.) Note to reader: The original legends have been included, to explain what the graphs are meant to show.

been "as our correspondent" (JAMA 100 Years Ago. JAMA 286;140). Today some major medical journals seem to have a monthly column correcting errors in recently published papers. Most errata are of minor significance, other than the damage to the self-esteem of the authors. Much more egregious, even dangerous, are errors involving drug doses. I recently received a copy of the 16th edition of the *Handbook of Antimicrobial Therapy* published by the Medical Letter on Drugs and Therapeutics. The handbook came with an attached warning label:

> On page 130 the pediatric dosage of doxycycline (combined with quinine sulfate) for treatment of chloroquine-resistant *P. falciparum* malaria should be 2 mg/kg/d × 7d.

On page 130 of the handbook, the dose is listed as 30 mg/kg/d × 7d. This is much more worrisome than incorrect fractions in a job advertisement.

After Publication

Saving Your Files
Some people save empty boxes, lengths of ribbon, odd pieces of wood, and half-empty cans of paint. They will tell you, "I might use this some day." Saving stuff is a very good idea for writers. I tend to file by project. I have a file with all the notes and quotes used for this book. If I plan to use something from this book in another project, I will make a copy for the new book or article. Items you liked, but didn't actually use, might be just what you need for your next article or book. For example, I have an idea for a new book that will be along the same lines as this one. When I come across papers or anecdotes that may be useful, I drop them in a file, unsorted for now. My files include metaphors, similes, and examples that might support one of my pet theories. I also keep a computer file of topic ideas that may become chapter titles or section headings. Some of these items accumulate for years, and then turn out to be useful. That is how I happen to have this chapter's reference 12 from 1985.

Reprints
Sometime during the production process, you will probably be asked whether you would like to purchase reprints of your

paper. Reprints are a time-honored tradition in scientific writing, and before the Internet were an important way in which investigators disseminated their findings.

A century ago, C. D. Spivak,[15] the editor of *Medical Libraries*, reported, "There is an inborn craving in the hearts of medical men for reprints of their articles." He attributed this craving to "a psychological fact, namely, that every writer wishes to give the stamp of individuality to his work." Spivak called for authors to let medical libraries be the first claimant on reprints.

Today, reprints seem to be going out of fashion, and I don't buy them anymore. They have become expensive. Journals use them to generate income, and seem unable to sell me a reasonably small number. I receive very few requests from individuals whom I know share my scientific interests. Most requests seem to be postcards from individuals in distant lands, whom I suspect request dozens of reprints monthly. Each year more and more journals go online, and I predict that in time journal reprints, like my file of journal clippings, will become a historical curiosity.

Criticism
There is an old aphorism about medical writing: He who writes stands up to be shot at. After publication of your article, chapter, or book, some readers may write letters to the editor saying, "Great job." (In fact, such letters are unlikely to be published, because they do not generate controversy.) Some book reviewers may praise your work. The first edition of my book *Family Medicine: Principles and Practice* was reviewed in the *British Medical Journal* as "the Cecil & Loeb/Gray's Anatomy of family practice for the foreseeable future." Wow! A quarter century later, I still feel good about this review. When you and I receive such accolades, we should enjoy them—because they are the exception.

Other book reviewers and letter writers have reported that I have misspelled words, "missed the mark," and, in one instance, was an example of why no single physician should be the sole author of a medical book. I have endured my share of harsh criticism.

The *New England Journal of Medicine* published a paper on the prevention of radiocontrast-agent–induced nephropathy by hemofiltration (Marenzi G, Marana I, Lauri G, et al. The prevention of radiocontrast-agent–induced nephropathy by hemofiltration. NEJM 2003;349:1333–1340). A response letter was published stating, "Several key points cast doubts on the conclusions drawn by Marenzi and colleagues" (Forman JP. Letter. NEJM 2004;350:837).

JAMA published a paper on treating ventilator-associated pneumonia (Chastre J, Wolff M, Fagon JY, et al. Comparison of 8 vs 15 days of antibiotic therapy for ventilator-associated pneumonia in adults: a randomized trial. JAMA 2003;290: 2588–2598). In response, a writer states, "I have some concerns about the design of this study" (Nicastri E. Letter. JAMA 2004;291:820).

The most serious criticism and editorial reaction I have noted recently were as follows. In 2001, the publishers of *Human Immunology* retracted an immunogenetics paper that some believed contained inappropriate content. Statements in the paper concerning culture, religion, and genetics ruffled political feathers. The journal editors deleted the article from the online edition of the journal and requested that medical librarians tear the article pages from their printed, often bound, issues of the journal.

The conclusion must be that as a medical writer you must have thick skin. All you can do is write your article or book chapter, check everything carefully, have the manuscript reviewed by a colleague, and then submit for publication. When the paper appears in print, be prepared to take the barbs, or perhaps the applause, that may come from readers and reviewers. Take pride in the fact that you have successfully navigated the review process and had your paper published, and that your critic has, in fact, been one of your readers.

BEYOND PUBLICATION

At the beginning of the chapter I mentioned that there are more steps after publication. Some of these possibilities are presented next.

Writing Teams, Support Groups, and Courses

I am a strong advocate of *writing teams* for beginning authors, especially when a research study is being planned. Writing teams pick a topic, select a leader, divide the work, and then meet regularly until the article is in print. The project becomes fun, and work moves forward because no one wants to let the group down.

The *writing support group* is composed of clinicians, and perhaps others, who are committed to improving their writing skills. There may be a group leader, or leadership may rotate. Generally one member presents his or her work, followed by criticism by others in the group. Sometimes the group uses specific writing exercises. Fundamentally these are support groups of persons who provide one another with encouragement, while allowing members to applaud one another's successes and grieve colleagues' rejections.

Grzybowski et al[16] describe a writing group at a hospital in Vancouver, Canada. The group met regularly over 3 years. Fifty writing projects were discussed, and 12 of those were subsequently published in indexed journals. The seven group members who attended most frequently saw an increase in their publication rate over 3 years of more than 300%.

In an academic setting, 18 assistant professors participated in a writing and faculty development program with seven monthly 75-minute sessions. By the end of the program, all participants completed at least one scholarly manuscript.[17] This activity seems to be both a writing course and a writers' support group.

Fellowships

Fellowships offer opportunities for clinicians who want to go further with their writing and editing. Here are three examples. All provide a modest stipend. If unsuccessful in reaching the e-mail address listed here, contact the journal's editorial office directly, after finding contact information using a Google search.

Morris Fishbein Fellowship in Medical Editing

Named in honor of a former editor of JAMA, this fellowship offers the opportunity to work with the journal's staff in all facets of editing and publishing a major medical journal. The fellow's work is supervised by a physician-editor, and as part of the duties, the fellow will be expected to prepare articles for publication. If interested, contact: richard_glass@jama-archives.org.

New England Journal of Medicine Editorial Fellow

This one-year position combines editorial experience with research. The fellow will participate in editorial and journal activities, but is expected to have his or her own independent projects. Applications, including a description of your research interests, should be mailed to: NEJM Editor-in-Chief, 10 Shattuck Road, Boston, MA 02115.

John C. Rose Fellowship

The *American Family Physician* (AFP) journal offers a year-long medical editing fellowship. This fellowship combines experiences in medical editing and writing with the opportunity to teach residents and medical students. Some patient care is required. The fellow works with the AFP editor, reviews manuscripts, writes items for the journal, and learns about the process of journal production. The contact address by e-mail is: siwekj@georgetown.edu.

Contests

Several journals sponsor writing contests. An example is the Creative Medical Writing Contest sponsored by the *Journal of General Internal Medicine* (JGIM). There are "prizes for the best submission in each of the categories of poetry or prose about the experience of being a patient, a patient's family member, a health-care provider, a medical researcher, or a student." The prize awards are modest, but winning submissions have a high probability of publication. If interested be sure to check with the JGIM about submission requirements. More information is available at: http://www.sgim.org/creativemedwrite.cfm.

The practicing clinician with writing skills and an interest in clinical issues should consider the *Medical Economics* writing contest. The 2003 grand prize was a $6000 vacation. If interested, contact the journal Web site or write to: Outside Copy Editor, Medical Economics, 5 Paragon Drive, Montvale, NJ 07645.

Contests are announced periodically and then have deadlines. Be sure to check for up-to-date information if considering a submission.

American Medical Writers Association

The American Medical Writers Association (AMWA), with approximately 5000 members, is the leading professional organization for biomedical communicators. Membership is open to all who write, edit, or teach about writing in areas such as medical science, biotechnology, or the pharmaceutical industry.

AMWA offers continuing professional education, which includes courses and workshops. Each quarter, the organization publishes the *AMWA Journal*, a source of information and opportunities in the field of biomedical communication. Some recent article topics in the journal were "The Ethical Challenges of Explaining Science" and "Common Statistical Errors Even YOU Can Find." If interested in learning more about AMWA, contact the organization at: amwa@amwa.org.

Self-Publication

Self-publication of an article, poem, or cartoon is easy. Just type the following at the bottom of the page: Copyright, your name, and the current year. Then print out the document, give it to a friend, and it is published. Legally no one can copy this now-published document without your permission. But this is not the topic of this section.

Many clinicians write books, and then they find that attaining publication is difficult. In fact, without an agent, it is almost impossible for the beginning writer to find a publisher for a trade book. Also, agents are busy and most won't read your book unless you are a published book author. Do you see the problem here? Clinical books, if timely and well written, are more likely to be published but this process can also be challenging. (See Chapter 8 and my advice never to write a book without a signed contract with a publisher.)

Nevertheless, let's assume that you are a clinician who has written a book. Perhaps your book is the great medical mystery novel, your heart-felt autobiography, or *How I Learned Neurosurgery on the Internet in Five Easy Lessons*. Sadly, no publisher has recognized the value and marketing potential of your book, and the manuscript is beginning to turn a little yellow.

Then you come across the magazine advertisement that reads, "AUTHORS WANTED, Leading subsidy book publisher seeks manuscripts. Fiction, non-fiction, poetry, juvenile, religious, etc. New authors welcome" (*Smithsonian Magazine*, February 2004, p. 103).

Perhaps you are surfing the Barnes and Noble Web site and come upon their Select program, which offers a contract, assistance with publishing, a custom cover, and quick availability. Your book will be ready for sale within 90 days. For each of these services you pay a fee, and you receive one or more copies of your book.

Self-publication, called subsidy publication, is the last refuge of the desperate author. The problem is distribution. There is no publishing company with an investment in your effort out there trying hard to sell your book, and you do not have the time or resources to do so. You will have copies to give your parents and your kids. You can show your book to your friends. You will almost certainly not make money on the transaction. Your satisfaction with the process will depend on your feelings about seeing your name and your work in print.

Years ago a friend and I acquired the translation of a book written overseas. It was a medical book for the lay public. We formed a corporation called Erbonia Books and published the book. We then owned a garage full of books. No one beat a path to our garage door to buy books. Several local bookstores stocked a few copies, as a favor to us, but sales were sparse. We ran magazine advertisements, but none brought enough orders to cover the cost of the advertisements. Eventually we were lucky; my partner had a friend who worked for a major publishing firm in New York City. This company bought the rights to our book and published a paperback edition that finally had national distribution. When all was said and done, we spent a lot of time and effort. Our original printing costs and advertising costs exceeded the royalties received from the real publisher. We had learned a lesson, and we disincorporated Erbonia Books.

I am not a fan of self-publication.

PUTTING IT ALL TOGETHER

Medical articles and book chapters traditionally have a "summary" section at the end. This is it.

A Word from the Author

When you go to live theater, you get something from the performance and you give something to the actors, musician, and writers. I believe that something like this happens when reading an article or, in this instance, a book. In writing this book, I have offered my best advice and most clever personal stories. In return you have given your attention, especially if you have reached this page in your reading. In doing so, you allow me to assume that I may be some small help in your future writing successes. For me, that is the real reward of the writing effort.

Remember that writing is a continuous process. The writer does not think about the writing episodically. For a writer, the current task, and maybe the next, will always be lurking in the subconscious mind. You will be sensitive to the analogy, the anecdote, and the image that can make your work sparkle just a little. Writing does not occur just when you turn on your computer. The mining of your personal experience and connectivity, cataloging ideas and images, and organizing ideas are all part of writing.

In the 1987 movie titled *Throw Momma from the Train*, Billy Crystal plays a down-on-his-luck English literature teacher leading an adult night school course in creative writing. Danny DeVito plays a not-too-bright student aspiring to be a writer. At several key points in the movie, Crystal emphasizes to DeVito, "A writer writes!" In the end, both successfully publish their books.

I urge you to join me and others in writing. See it as an ongoing journey of education, self-discovery, and personal growth. For me, writing this book has been part of such a process. I hope that you have enjoyed reading it half as much as I have enjoyed writing it. I am sorry to see it end. But I have another project in mind to start next week.

My last offering in the book is a personal indulgence. We have all heard of Robert's Rules of Order. Here are Doctor Taylor's Rules for Medical Writers:

- *Be smart enough*. Yet, be well aware that being intelligent is not enough.
- *Be organized*. Keep files and notes, with full reference citations, whether on paper or computer. Know where things are, and take the time needed to systematize all your writing materials.
- *Be a reader*. Always be reading something, and seek a wide range of topics. While reading, note both what is said and how the author expresses the ideas.
- *Be a good time-manager*. Clinical care is your day job, and it cannot be neglected. Patients will suffer and you will lose your wellspring of writing ideas. But you must also carve out regular, dependable time for writing if you are ever to finish a project.
- *Be an effective networker*. Get to know medical editors, other writers, and—if planning to edit a multiauthor book— potential authors. Make the ongoing effort needed to nurture these relationships.
- *Be bold*. Don't hesitate to aim high or to propose the project that seems beyond your abilities. Those who take on too much, with too little time and too few resources, sometimes succeed.
- *Be persistent*. Writers endure rejection often. You must be able to bounce back and revise and resubmit or even start over. But you must not give up on your writing. A writer writes.

Now it's time to Write It Up. Have fun!

REFERENCES

1. King LS. Why not say it clearly? Boston: Little, Brown; 1978:5.
2. Callaham M, Wears RL, Weber E. Journal prestige, publication bias, and other characteristics associated with citation of published studies in peer-reviewed journals. JAMA 2002;287: 2847–2850.
3. Norton SA. Read this but skip that. J Am Acad Dermatol 2001;44:714–715.
4. Grouse LD. A rogue's gallery of medical manuscripts. JAMA 1980;244:700–701.
5. von Elm D, Poglia G, Walder B, Tramer MR. Different patterns of duplicate publication: an analysis of articles used in systematic reviews. JAMA 2004;291:974–980.
6. International Committee of Medical Journal Editors. Uniform Requirements for manuscripts submitted to biomedical journals. Updated October 2001. http://www.icmje.org.
7. The New England Journal of Medicine. Instructions for submission. http://www.nejm.org/hfa/subinstr.asp.
8. Academic Medicine. Instructions for authors. http://www.academicmedicine.org/misc/ifora.shtml.
9. Whimster WF. Biomedical research; how to plan, publish and present it. New York: Springer-Verlag; 1997:136, 149.
10. PaperTRAIL—Paper TRAcking through Interactive Links for the New England Journal of Medicine. http://www.nejm.org/hfa/papertrail/.
11. Kübler-Ross E. On death and dying. New York: Macmillan; 1969.
12. Strasburger VC. Righting medical writing. JAMA 1985;254: 1789–1790.
13. Coates R, Sturgeon B, Bohannan J, Pasini E. Language and publication in "Cardiovascular Research" articles. Cardiovasc Res 2002;53(2):279–285.
14. Peters DP, Ceci SJ. Peer-review practices of psychological journals: the fate of published articles, submitted again. Behav Brain Sci 1982;5:187–255.
15. Spivak CD. Reprints, whence they come and whither they should go. JAMA 2002;287:1911.
16. Grzybowski SC, Bates J, Calam B, et al. A physician peer support writing group. Fam Med 2003;35(3):195–201.
17. Pololi L, Knight S, Dunn K. Facilitating scholarly writing in academic medicine: lessons learned from a collaborative peer-mentoring program. J Gen Intern Med 2004;19(1):64–68.

Appendix 1. Glossary of Terms Used in Medical Writing

Author   Someone who actively participated in preparation of a paper or book, and who assumes intellectual responsibility for its content.

Boolean logic   An approach to relationships among search terms, using AND, OR, and NOT (named for George Boole, mathematician).

Camera-ready copy   Material, generally figures, that do not require typesetting and are suitable for photographic reproduction as submitted. Complicated chemical structures and mathematical formulas are generally best submitted as camera-ready copy.

Caption   See Legend.

Career topic   The topic that you present in writing and in lectures throughout your career, keeping up with all advances in the field. For clinicians, this is most likely to be a disease (such as hypertension), a clinical presentation (such as chest pain), or a procedure (such as retinal surgery or minimally invasive management of breast cancer).

Compositor   The person who sets the type for your article as it is being prepared for printing. A synonym is typesetter, although technically type is no longer "set."

Copyeditor   The person who makes needed improvements in grammar and syntax, and then marks up a manuscript for the printer. The copyeditor is generally employed by the publisher, and often is the author's "best friend."

Copyright   The legal right to publish, copy, sell, or otherwise use a specific intellectual property.

Editor   The editor holds the powerful position of deciding which manuscripts are published and which "do not meet our publication needs at this time." There are also various types of editor, especially in book publishing: acquisition editors, development editors, production editors, associate editors, and copyeditors.

Electronic journal An online version of a medical publication. At this time, most electronic medical journals are extensions of print publications. In the future, there are likely to be many freestanding electronic journals.

Galley proofs, galleys A copy of typeset matter, usually printed in columns, intended to be reviewed by the author before being made into page proofs.

Halftone A figure composed of shades of gray, usually a "black and white" photograph or a shaded drawing.

Impact factor The total number of citations made for a journal in a year for articles published in two previous years divided by the number of citable articles published in these years. It is used to judge the quality of a journal. See Chapter 5.

IMRAD An acronym that represents the organizational structure most often used in research reports: Introduction, Methods, Results, and Discussion. See Chapter 9.

Legend Also sometimes called a "caption," the legend is the title of a figure or table, and may also provide explanatory information.

Line drawing, line art A figure composed of black and white lines, such as a graph, diagram, or drawing that is not shaded.

Loansome Doc A feature in PubMed that allows the user to place an electronic order through the National Network of Libraries of Medicine for the full-text copy of an article found on MEDLINE.

Mark-up This refers to both the process and the symbols by which copyeditors communicate specific instructions to typesetters.

MDConsult A subscription-based Web site that allows one to search medical reference books, medical journals, MEDLINE, and drug information. Includes clinical practice guidelines and patient education handouts: www.mdconsult.com.

MEDLINE (Medical Literature, Analysis, and Retrieval System Online) The U.S. National Library of Medicine's (NLM) leading bibliographic database. It contains more than 12 million references to journal articles in the life sciences, chiefly in biomedicine. It can be searched via PubMed or the NLM gateway: www.nlm.nih.gov.

MeSH (Medical Subject Headings) The National Library of Medicine's controlled vocabulary thesaurus. It consists of sets of terms that permit searching MEDLINE at various levels of specificity.

Meta-analysis A method of combining the results of several studies into a summary conclusion, using quantitative strategies that will allow consideration of data in diverse research reports.

Monograph A specialized book, usually relatively short and generally written by one or a small group of medical specialists.

National Library of Medicine The world's largest medical library with collections in all major areas of the health sciences, and the home of MEDLINE and PubMed.

Network research The process of using sequential contacts to find out a needed fact. The key question in network research is, "Who do you recommend that I call next?" For more details, see Chapter 3.

Offprints See Reprints.

Overlay A transparent sheet with graphic material to be superimposed on another page.

Page proofs A copy of typeset text laid out as it will appear in print, including headings and page numbers.

Pagination The process of numbering the pages of a manuscript. Your word processing program can do this for you.

Peer review, peer reviewer The evaluation of a submitted manuscript by individuals with like credentials, usually performed without the peer reviewers knowing who wrote the manuscript or the author knowing who performed the review. Peer reviewers may also be called referees.

Proof A copy of a work that has been set in type, sent to authors or editors to review for errors. Proof may be galley proofs, when not yet set as pages, or may be actual page proofs of the article or book pages.

Proofreader's marks A set of symbols used to identify errors or changes on proofs. See Appendix 2.

PubMed A Web site that is a service of the National Library of Medicine, with more than 14 million citations for biomedical articles from MEDLINE and other sources. PubMed is discussed in Chapter 1, and can be accessed at http://www.pubmed.com.

Redaction The process of word-by-word, sentence-by-sentence modification of a paper.

Referee See Peer review.

Reprints Also sometimes called "offprints," these are separately printed copies of individual journal articles. Journals generally provide these to authors for a fee.

Research report Also called a "scientific paper," the research report discusses the results of a research study.

Review article A paper that deals with known information in a thoughtful way, but does not present the results of a clinical research study.

Running head A shorthand listing of items—usually an abbreviated title of the article that appears at the top of each page. It allows the editor to reassemble the manuscript if it is blown about by the wind. Because of the anonymity of peer review, most journals do not want author names included in the running head.

Science Citation Index (SCI) A proprietary database of citations of published articles, it is also used to calculate the journal impact factor.

Stop A unit of punctuation that breaks the flow of words. Stops include the comma, colon, semicolon, question mark, and exclamation mark.

Target journal   As you prepare an article, the target journal is number one on your list of publication possibilities. This is where you would like your article published, and the article's format and style should mirror those of the target journal.

Tear sheets   Pages removed from a previously published book, generally used when revising an edition of the book.

Trade books   Books published to be sold to the general public, not to the market of professional clinicians. Books for clinicians and other scholars are called professional books.

Typesetting   The process of composing the edited manuscript as it will appear in the final pages.

Uniform Requirements for Manuscripts Submitted to Biomedical Journals   A statement available on the Web that states how to prepare a paper for a medical journal. It also covers statements on related ethical issues in research and writing. See further discussion in Chapter 1. Access the latest version at: www.icmje.org.

UpToDate   A subscription-based Web site that provides topic reviews on clinical topics: http://www.uptodate.com.

Validity   The extent to which a study measures what it was intended to measure.

Appendix 2. Commonly Used Proofreader's Marks

The following symbols are used when correcting galley and page proofs.

Mark the text	In the margin	Meaning
Now is ⓘs the time	ℓ	Delete; take out
Now is the ti̭me	⌒	Close up
Now is the ti̭a̭me	ℯ̂	Delete and close up
Nowis the time	#	Insert space
Now∧ is the time	ℓℊ #	Equal space between words
Now∧the time	is	Insert word(s)
It is time∧We	⊙	Insert period
It is time∧but	∧	Insert comma
It is time∧we	;	Insert semicolon
High∧energy pump	⌒	Insert hyphen
Smith∧1977∧ stated	(/)/	Insert parentheses
Smith₃ statement	⌣	Insert apostrophe
Evaluation of ln e∧	⋎	Insert as superscript
The value of Ḙmax	max	Make subscript
the vᵃlue	≡	Straighten line(s)
all cases.∧The value⌐	¶	Make new paragraph
⌐of most data …	no ¶	No paragraph – run in
Teh of value is	(tr.) //	Transpose
⊏E_max	⊏	Move left as indicated
E_max ⊐	⊐	Move right as indicated
now is the time	cap	Capital
Smith (1977) said	s.c.	Small capitals
Now is The time	l.c.	Lower case
Now is the time	Rom	Roman type
Now is the time	ital	Italic
now is the time	cap ital	Capital italic
Now is the time	bf	Boldface type
S_sp (1977) stated	sp	Spell out
Now is the time	stet	Let stand as is

Appendix 3. Commonly Used Medical Abbreviations*

Abbreviation	Meaning
ACE	Angiotensin-converting enzyme
ACTH	Adrenocorticotropic hormone
AIDS	Acquired immunodeficiency syndrome
ALT	Alanine aminotransferase (SGPT)
ANA	Antinuclear antibody
AST	Aspartate aminotransferase (SGOT)
bid	Twice a day
BP	Blood pressure
bpm	Beats per minute
BS	Blood sugar
BUN	Blood urea nitrogen
CBC	Complete blood count
CHF	Congestive heart failure
Cl^-	Chloride
CO_2	Carbon dioxide
COPD	Chronic obstructive pulmonary disease
CPR	Cardiopulmonary resuscitation
CSF	Cerebrospinal fluid
CT	Computed tomography
cu mm	Cubic millimeter
CXR	Chest x-ray
d	Day, daily
dL	Deciliter
DM	Diabetes mellitus
ECG	Electrocardiogram
ESR	Erythrocyte sedimentation rate
FDA	United States Food and Drug Administration
g	Gram

* May be used in your medical writing. No specific permission form is required for use. Please give full credit to this book as the source.

GI	Gastrointestinal
Hb	Hemoglobin
Hg	Mercury
HIV	Human immunodeficiency virus
HMO	Health maintenance organization
hr	Hour
hs	Hours of sleep, at bedtime
HTN	Hypertension
IM	Intramuscular
INR	International normalized ratio
IU	International unit
IV	Intravenous
K^+	Potassium
kg	Kilogram
L	Liter
LD or LDH	Lactate dehydrogenase
mEq	Milliequivalent
μg	Microgram
mg	Milligram
min	Minute
mL	Milliliter
mm	Millimeter
mm^3	Cubic millimeter
MRI	Magnetic resonance imaging
Na^+	Sodium
NSAID	Nonsteroidal antiinflammatory drug
po	By mouth *(per os)*
PT	Prothrombin time
PTT	Partial thromboplastin time
q	Every
qd	Every day; daily
qid	Four times a day
qod	Every other day
RBC	Red blood cell, red blood count
SC	Subcutaneous
sec	Second
SGOT	See AST
SGPT	See ALT
STD	Sexually transmitted disease
TB	Tuberculosis

tid	Three times a day
TSH	Thyroid-stimulating hormone
U	Unit
UA	Urine analysis
WBC	White blood cell, white blood count

Appendix 4. Normal Laboratory Values for Adult Patients*

CLINICAL CHEMISTRY TESTS

Alanine aminotransferase (ALT, SGPT)	0–35 U/L
Albumin	3.6–5.2 g/dL
Alkaline phosphatase (ALP)	35–120 U/L
Amylase, serum	44–128 U/L
Aspartate aminotransferase (AST, SGOT)	0–35 U/L
Bilirubin, conjugated	0–0.2 mg/dL
Bilirubin, total	0.2–1.2 mg/dL
Calcium	8.5–10.5 mg/dL
Carbon dioxide (CO_2), total	23–30 mEq/L
Chloride	98–109 mEq/L
Creatine kinase (CK, CPK)	30–170 U/L
Creatinine	0.7–1.2 mg/dL
Gamma glutamyltransferase (GGT)	5–40 U/L
Glucose, fasting	65–110 mg/dL
Hemoglobin A_{1C}	5.0–7.0% of total Hb
Iron, serum	50–170 µg/dL
Iron binding capacity, total (TIBC)	270–390 µg/dL
Lactate, serum (venous)	5.0–20.0 mg/dL
Lactate dehydrogenase (LDH)	110–260 U/L
Lipase	10–140 U/L
Magnesium	1.5–2.5 mg/dL
Potassium	3.5–5.1 mEq/L
Prostate-specific antigen	0–4 ng/mL
Protein, total	6.1–7.9 g/dL
Sodium	136–147 mEq/L

* May be used in your medical writing. No specific permission form is required for use. Please give full credit to this book as the source.

Troponin I	<2.5 ng/mL
Troponin T	<0.2 ng/mL
Urea nitrogen	6.0–23.0 mg/dL
Uric acid	2.6–7.2 mg/dL

LIPID PANEL

Cholesterol, total	160–240 mg/dL
HDL cholesterol	>40 mg/dL
LDL cholesterol	<130 mg/dL
Triglycerides	55–200 mg/dL

THYROID FUNCTION TESTS

Thyroid stimulating hormone (TSH)	2–11 μU/mL
Thyroxine, free (FT_4)	0.8–2.4 ng/dL
Thyroxine, total (T_4)	4.0–12.0 μg/dL
Triiodothyronine (T_3)	70–200 ng/dL
Triiodothyronine (T_3) resin uptake (T_3 RU)	25–38%

BLOOD GASES

	Arterial	*Venous*
Base excess	-3.0 to $+3.0$ mEq/L	-5.0 to $+5.0$ mEq/L
Bicarbonate (HCO_3)	18–25 mEq/L	18–25 mEq/L
pO_2	80–95 mm Hg	30–48 mm Hg
O_2 saturation	95–98%	60–85%
pCO_2	34–45 mm Hg	35–52 mm Hg
Total CO_2	23–30 mEq/L	24–31 mEq/L
pH	7.35–7.45	7.32–7.42

HEMATOLOGY AND COAGULATION TESTS

White cell (WBC) count	3.4–10.0 K/mm^3
Hemoglobin	12.2–18.0 g/dL
Hematocrit	37.0–54.0%
Red cell (RBC) count	3.80–5.20 million/mm^3
Mean corpuscular volume (MCV)	85.0–95.0 μm^3

Mean corpuscular hemoglobin (MCH)	26.0–34.0 pg/cell
MCH concentration (MCHC)	32.6–36.0 g/dL
Red cell distribution width (RDW)	11.5–15.0%
Platelet count	150.0–420.0 K/mm^3
Reticulocyte count	0.5–1.5% of RBCs
WBC differential	
Neutrophils	38–70%
Lymphocytes	16–49%
Monocytes	2–9%
Eosinophils	0–5%
Basophils	0–2%
Sedimentation rate	
Adult male	≤ 15 mm/h
Adult female	≤ 20 mm/h
Coagulation tests	
Fibrinogen	200–400 mg/dL
Partial thromboplastin time (PTT)	60–85 seconds
Activated PTT	25–35 seconds
Prothrombin time (PT)	11–14 seconds

Note: The reference intervals shown are for adults, and may vary according to technique or laboratory or as new methods are introduced. Always consult the reference range for your own laboratory.

Index

Abbreviations 115–116, 255–257
Abstract 201–202
Acceptance letter 230
Acceptance rate 231
  author recruitment 183
  journals 24, 215
Accuracy and precision 113–115
Acquisitions editor 179
Acronyms 117
Adjectives 53–54
Advances 181
Adverbs 53–54
Affiliations 152, 231
Algorithms 95–96
Alliteration 55
Alternative words and
  constructions 75–76
American Medical Writers
  Association 241
Article submission 213–214
Audience 23–24, 57, 111, 129–132
Author
  agreement 183
  ghost 122–123
  honorary 122–123
  recruitment 182–183
  reminders 184
Authored books 168, 188–191, *see
  also* Edited books
Authorship 120

Barriers to writing 4–6
Book chapters
  agreements 170–171, 172
  invitation to write 168–170
  preparing and submitting
    172–173
  structure 173–175
  submitting 175–176
Book proposal 180–181

Book reviews 25–26, 155–162
  how to write 158–160
  types of 156–157
  warnings about 162
  what makes a good 161–162
Boolean searching 18, 247
Borrowed materials 98–102

Cadence 45
Camera-ready copy 88, 96, 103, 247
Case reports 25, 89, 109, 143–146,
    148, 153, 154, 214
  format 145–146
  types of 145
Clarity 74–75
Colleague as a critical reader 81–82
Commas 46
Complementary copies 155, 169,
    181–182, 190
Compositor 247
Computer 13–14
Computer programs 16–17
Concept 61–63
Conflict of interest 120–121
Contests 240–241
Contract 181–182
Copyediting 62–63, 187, 232, 234
Copyeditor 247
Copyright 97–98, 99, 247
Courses 239
Creativity 10–11
Critical argument 149
Critical review 81–82
Criticism 237–238
Cuteness 80
Cutting material 77–79

Data, collecting and organizing 63–68
Delaying tactics 70
Development editor 184

Dictionaries 14–15, 16
Draft
  final 82–83
  first 68–72
Drug references 15, 17

Edited books 167–168, 176–188
  compiling 184–186
  initiating 176–177
  planning 177–178
  publication 186–187
Editor 247–248
Editorials 25, 30, 146–150, 152, 214
  preparation 149–150
  types of 147–149
Electronic journal 248
EMBASE 109
Enrichment books 167
Eponyms 55–56
Errors 57, 81, 82, 87, 88, 96, 113,
    114–115, 122, 140, 158, 160,
    178, 187, 188, 207, 222, 231,
    233, 234–236, *see also*
    Grammar, errors
Ethical issues 120–123
Evidence-based clinical review
    138–140
Expertise 30, 148–149

Fellowships 239–240
Figures 88–97
Files, saving 236

Getting stuck 70–72
Google search engine 18
Gorging 112
Grammar
  errors 62, 73, 187, 232
  tools 42, 222
  use of tense 40–42
  see also specific terms
Graphs 92–94
Grazing 111–112

Halftones 90–91, 248
History
  of medicine articles 163
  role of medical writing 7–8

Hubris 123
Hunting 112

Idea development 29–32
Impact rating, *see* Journal Impact
    Factor
IMRAD model of research reports
    198, 248
Index Medicus 109, 203
Informal refereeing, *see* Critical
    review
Institute for Scientific Information
    (ISI) 109
International Committee of Medical
    Journal Editors (ICMJE) 106
Internet 6, 13, 19
  security 13–14

Jargon 113, 114
Journal editors 134, 215–216
  possible responses from 226–230
  role and duties 225
Journal Impact Factor 109–111,
    214–215
Journals
  broad-based peer-reviewed
      106–107
  controlled-circulation 107
  indexing 108–109
  online 108
  specialty oriented peer-reviewed
      107
  types of 106–108

Key words 202–203

Legend 248
Letters to the editor 25, 104, 150–155
  types of 151–153
  writing 153–155
Line drawings 91–92, 248
Literature review update 220
Litigation 152
Loansome Doc 248

Mailing 222
Mark-up 248
Market rules 192–193

MDConsult 20, 248
Medical books, types of 167
Medical publication opportunities, miscellaneous 162, 163
MEDLINE/PubMed 19–20, 109, 249, 250
Mentors 210
MeSH (Medical Subject Headings) 249
Meta-analysis 137, 249
Metaphors 54–55
Mistakes
  when starting 26
  in structuring 35–36
  see also Errors
Modifiers 53–54
Monograph 249
Movie reviews 164

National Library of Medicine (NLM) 19, 249
Native language 231
Network research 63–64, 249
Newspaper columns 165–166
Notes 64–65
Nouns 52–53

Offprints 249
Onomatopoeia 55
Outlines 33–34, 65–67
Overlay 249
Overstatement 123

Packing 222
Page proofs 249
Pagination 249
Paragraph
  development 36–40
  examples 38–39
  organizing 37–38
Peer review 230–231, 249
Peer reviewers 24, 81, 107, 121, 127, 143, 215, 216, 223, 229, 249
  role and duties 224–225
Periods 47
Permissions 98–102
Personal relationships 193
Photographs, *see* Halftones

Plagiarism 122
Planning 34, 177–178
Poetry 162–163
Postpublication 188
Practice tips 165
Professional books 191–192
Profile of a writer 10
Project-specific industry support 121
Pronouns 52–53
Proof 250
Proofreader's marks 250, 253
Proofreading 232–234
Publisher, finding potential 179
PubMed, *see* MEDLINE/PubMed
Punctuation 45–49

Question marks 47
Questions 164
Quizes 163

Reader consideration 39–40
Reading
  for ideas 8–9
  for information 8–9
  for style 9–10
  for writing 2–4
Red-flag phrases 79
Redaction 250
Referees 250, *see also* Peer reviewers
Reference books 14–16, 167
Reference citations 102–104
References 67–68
Rejection 2, 24, 27, 81, 83, 103, 153, 215, 216, 223, 225, 226–229, 244
  letters 226–229
  causes of 227
Reprints 236–237, 250
Research reports 250
  acknowledgments 209
  authors 200
  careers and 211
  discussion 207
  introduction 203–204
  methods 205
  references 208
  results 206–207
  title 199

Resources 12–22, 63–64
Review article 250
 definition 127–128
 planning 132–134
 publishers of 128–129, 130–131
 readership 129–132
 special types 135–140
 structure 133
 see also Meta-analysis, Evidence-
  based clinical review
Review journal
 consulting editor 134
 errors when writing for 140–141
Review process 223–232
Revision 72–82
 letter 229
Royalties 3, 169, 181, 192
Running head 250

Science Citation Index (SCI) 250
Self-publication 241–243
Semicolons 46
Sentence density 44
Sentences 40–49
 active versus passive voice 40–42
 construction 42–45
 variety in 43
Similes 54–55
Skill of medical writing 1–2
Spell checker 16–17, 42–53, 73,
  222–223
Stance 123–124
Stop 250
Structure 32–36, 61–63, 173–175
Style 74–75
Submission
 assembly 220–221
 letter 218–219
Success 26–27, 118, 128–129, 160,
  173, 197, 228, 243
Support groups 239

Tables 85–88
Target journal 251
Tear sheets 251
Textbooks 191–192

Thesaurus 16
Title 32, 44, 86, 111–112, 116, 125,
  135–136, 199
 page 220
Tools, *see* Resources
Topic
 career 247
 focused 32, 33–34, 63
Trade books 191–192, 251
Typesetting 251

Understatement 123–124
Uniform Requirements for
  Manuscripts Submitted to
  Biomedical Journals 21–22,
  251
UpToDate 20–21, 251

Validity 251
Verbosity 47
Verbs 53
Verification 103–104

Waffling 123–124
Websites 17–22, 64, 99, 139, 150
 citation 208
 online journals 108
 publishers 179
 tracking manuscript progress 226
Word selection 75, 76
Words 49–59
 annoying 57–58
 choosing 56–57
 medical 49–51
 misused 58–59
 per sentence 42
 per verb 43
 types 52–56
Workshops 2, 5, 241
World Wide Web 6
Writing area 13–14
Writing models for beginners 24–26
Writing teams 239
 guidelines 118–119
 problems 119–120
Writing topics 11–12